Ethics and Professionalism in Healthcare

Recent social developments, such as demographic change, skill shortages and new medical technologies, have necessitated a transition in the traditional roles of healthcare professions. New forms of division of labour and interprofessional healthcare education are emerging while, at the same time, ethical challenges, such as corruption and conflicts of interest, have to be mastered.

This book addresses historical, conceptual and empirical aspects of professionalism and inter-professionalism in healthcare from an international and interdisciplinary perspective. The work is divided into five sections: historical and societal aspects of healthcare professions; learning and teaching healthcare professionalism; transformation of healthcare professions; professional leadership and team decision-making in healthcare; and ethical challenges to healthcare professionalism. The final chapter integrates the main ideas and perspectives on healthcare professionalism which have been developed throughout the book and highlights how the work in the diverse disciplines is interrelated.

The book will be a valuable reference for the many researchers and students with an interest in medical ethics, professionalism and comparative systems of healthcare.

Sabine Salloch is a Researcher in Medical Ethics at the Institute for Medical Ethics and History of Medicine, Ruhr-University Bochum, Germany. Her research interests include end-of-life decision-making, medical professionalism and bioethical methodology.

Verena Sandow is a Researcher in Medical Ethics and Applied Ethics at the Institute for Medical Ethics and History of Medicine, Ruhr-University Bochum, Germany. She works in the field of human medical research and research ethics.

Jan Schildmann is a Medical Ethicist and Physician. He is Researcher at the Institute for Medical Ethics and History of Medicine, Ruhr-University Bochum, Germany. His research covers topics in clinical ethics (i.e. end-of-life decisions, ethics support services), research ethics (i.e. personalised medicine, conflict of interest) and methodological aspects of empirical medical ethics.

Jochen Vollmann is Professor and Director at the Institute for Medical Ethics and History of Medicine and Chair of the Centre for Medical Ethics, Ruhr-University Bochum, Germany. Professor Vollmann's research interests include informed consent and capacity assessment, mental health ethics, end-of-life decision-making, advance directives, personalised medicine, medical professionalism, clinical ethics committees and clinical ethics consultation.

Ethics and Professionalism in Healthcare

Transition and challenges

Edited by

**Sabine Salloch, Verena Sandow,
Jan Schildmann, Jochen Vollmann**

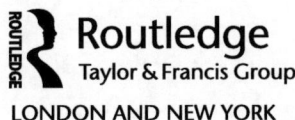

Routledge
Taylor & Francis Group

LONDON AND NEW YORK

First published 2016
by Routledge

2 Park Square, Milton Park, Abingdon, Oxfordshire OX14 4RN
52 Vanderbilt Avenue, New York, NY 10017

Routledge is an imprint of the Taylor & Francis Group, an informa business

First issued in paperback 2020

British Library Cataloguing-in-Publication Data
A catalogue record for this book is available from the British Library

Library of Congress Cataloging in Publication Data
Names: Salloch, Sabine, editor. | Sandow, Verena, editor. | Schildmann, Jan,
1974– , editor. | Vollmann, Jochen, editor.
Title: Ethics and professionalism in healthcare : transition and challenges /
edited by Sabine Salloch, Verena Sandow, Jan Schildmann and Jochen
Vollmann.
Description: Surrey, England ; Burlington, VT : Ashgate, [2016] | Includes
bibliographical references and index.
Identifiers: LCCN 2015043715 (print) | LCCN 2015047051 (ebook) |
ISBN 9781472479518 (hardback : alk. paper) | ISBN 9781472479525 (ebook) |
ISBN 9781472479532 (epub)
Subjects: | MESH: Ethics, Clinical. | Delivery of Health Care—ethics. |
Professional Role.
Classification: LCC R724 (print) | LCC R724 (ebook) | NLM WB 60 |
DDC 174.2—dc23
LC record available at http://lccn.loc.gov/2015043715

ISBN: 978-1-4724-7951-8 (hbk)
ISBN: 978-0-367-59644-6 (pbk)

Typeset in Bembo
by Keystroke, Station Road, Codsall, Wolverhampton

Contents

List of figures   ix
List of tables   xi
List of boxes   xiii
Notes on contributors   xv

1 **Introduction**   1
   SABINE SALLOCH, VERENA SANDOW, JAN SCHILDMANN
   AND JOCHEN VOLLMANN

PART I
Historical and societal aspects of healthcare professions   7

2 **A shifting focus from patients to employees:**
   withdrawal of religious communities and the
   emergence of political activity in Protestant hospitals
   in Berlin between 1960 and 1990   9
   CLEMENS TANGERDING

3 **How to write a letter: a physician's letters from the**
   viewpoint of medical humanities   25
   KATHARINA FÜRHOLZER

PART II
Learning and teaching healthcare professionalism   37

4 **Collaborative decision-making: a normative**
   synthesis of decision-making models in healthcare   39
   SARAH BERGER, CORNELIA MAHLER, JOBST-HENDRIK
   SCHULTZ, JOACHIM SZECSENYI AND KATJA GÖTZ

5 The Regensburg Model ('Pain Care Manager'): an
integrated interprofessional pain curriculum for
healthcare professionals in German-speaking countries   52
KIRSTIN FRAGEMANN, NICOLE LINDENBERG,
BERNHARD M. GRAF AND CHRISTOPH H. R. WIESE

PART III
Transformation of healthcare professions   71

6 Professionalism of the health workforce in Ukraine   73
TETIANA STEPURKO, ALONA GOROSHKO AND PAOLO CARLO BELLI

7 Transformation of the role of healthcare ethics
committees and the concept of clinical ethics in
Belarus: implications for medical professionalism   89
ANDREI FAMENKA

8 Ethical problems concerning the international brain
drain of healthcare professionals   101
DORINA MARIA STĂNESCU

PART IV
Professional leadership and team decision-making
in healthcare   111

9 Substituted or supported decisions? Examining
models of decision-making within interprofessional
team decision-making for individuals at risk of
lacking decision-making capacity   113
GEMMA CLARKE, SARAH GALBRAITH, JEREMY WOODWARD,
ANTHONY HOLLAND AND STEPHEN BARCLAY

10 Attitudinal, motivational and behavioural correlates
of ethical leadership in healthcare teams   126
MARTINA ŠENDULA-PAVELIĆ, ZORAN SUŠANJ AND ANA JAKOPEC

11 Cooperation between managers and the medical
profession in the context of strategic decision-making
in non-profit hospitals: a manageable challenge?   138
STEPHANIE RÜSCH

PART V
Ethical challenges to healthcare professionalism   149

12 **Akrasia and obedience in medicine: deferring to authority in a decision you believe to be wrong**   151
TIM WRAY, CHRISTOPHER YU AND CHRISTOPHER PHILBEY

13 **Professionalism in public health medicine and policy: the challenge of enhancement**   162
ALEX McKEOWN

14 **Ethics and professionalism in healthcare – a position paper**   178
SARAH BERGER, ANDREI FAMENKA, KIRSTIN FRAGEMANN,
KATHARINA FÜRHOLZER, ALEX McKEOWN,
STEPHANIE RÜSCH, MARTINA ŠENDULA-PAVELIĆ,
DORINA MARIA STĂNESCU, TETIANA STEPURKO,
CLEMENS TANGERDING AND CHRISTOPHER YU

Figures

5.1 Curricular interfaces of healthcare professions in pain
  management   59
5.2 Overview of course structure and course contents   61
5.3 Collaboration and satisfaction about care decisions
  (CSACD)   63
5.4 Participants' overall satisfaction as shown by course
  evaluation   65
11.1 Professional bureaucracy according to Mintzberg
  (1980)   140

Tables

5.1 Adapted version of the 'Knowledge and Attitudes
Survey Regarding Pain'   64

9.1 Model of decision-making axes upon which clinical
information was weighted to make decisions   118

9.2 Model of the process of FIMPT decision-making
based on a three-month non-participant observation   119

10.1 Descriptive statistics and correlations of all variables
measured   130

11.1 Sample   141

Boxes

4.1 Collaborative decision-making – a hybrid model
for healthcare   42
5.1 Summary response of final evaluations regarding
the overall satisfaction with the course programme
(open comments)   66
5.2 Reflections of a physician (general practitioner)
from a written case report   66
6.1 Example of the sensitive questions asked in the study   76

Contributors

Stephen Barclay is a Medical Practitioner in Cambridge, where he works clinically in both General Practice and Palliative Care. His 2005 MD thesis from the University of Cambridge was entitled 'General Practitioner provision of Palliative Care in the United Kingdom'. He is University Senior Lecturer in General Practice and Palliative Care in the University of Cambridge School of Clinical Medicine, where he leads a research group that focuses on palliative and end-of-life care in primary care, with a particular interest in General Practitioner and District Nurse provision of care, end-of-life care conversations in cancer and non-cancer illness, decision-making concerning treatment cessation in advanced disease and medical student education in Palliative Care. He also leads the teaching of Palliative Care to Cambridge medical students and is a Bye-Fellow and Director of Studies for Clinical Medicine at Emmanuel College, Cambridge.

Paolo Carlo Belli is a Lead Economist with the Human Development Unit, ECA Region, and Sector Leader for the Human Development Programme in Ukraine, Belarus and Moldova. Dr Belli has been at the World Bank since May 2003. In his professional career at the World Bank he has led several projects, including the preparation and supervision of several large lending operations in India, Sri Lanka, Moldova and Ukraine. Before joining the bank, Dr Belli was teaching at the Harvard School of Public Health, and before that he held a tenured academic position in Italy. Dr Belli has a PhD in Economics and Public Policy from the London School of Economics. In his academic career, Dr Belli has contributed to several research publications and initiatives, mainly in the areas of improving public sector management, health financing and governance.

Sarah Berger is a New Zealand Registered Nurse and lectures in the Bachelor of Science – Interprofessional Health Care at the Medical Faculty, University of Heidelberg. Her Master of Nursing (Honours) is from the University of Sydney, Australia, and her Master of Business Administration (MBA) and Bachelor of Arts (Philosophy and Literature) are from the University of Canterbury, New Zealand. Since 2012, she has held a research position at the Department of General Practice and Health Services

Research, University Hospital Heidelberg. She is currently working on her doctoral thesis on the subject of 'Structures and processes of ethical decision-making among health care students in an interprofessional education setting'. Other research interests include professionalism in health-care, regulatory frameworks, codes of conduct/ethics and interprofessional collaboration.

Gemma Clarke is a Research Associate in the Department of Public Health and Primary Care at the University of Cambridge. She is a social scientist with particular interests in eating and drinking issues at the end of life, and decision-making capacity. Currently, she leads the Future Care Study within the Palliative and End of Life Care Group. The Future Care Study is a project examining care and feeding issues at the end of life for those with progressive neurological disease, with and without decision-making capacity. Previously, she has worked on studies examining decision-making concerning artificial nutrition for those at risk of lacking capacity, and decisions to stop oral palliative anticancer drugs. In 2015, Gemma spent a term working in the USA as a visiting researcher at the Kennedy Institute of Ethics, Georgetown University in Washington, DC. Before joining the Department of Public Health and Primary Care, Gemma completed her PhD at the Institute of Criminology, Gonville and Caius College and worked as a Research Assistant at King's College London on the study, 'Young people and the secure estate: needs and interventions'. Gemma holds a Research Associateship at Homerton College, Cambridge.

Andrei Famenka is a Legal Medicine specialist at the Legal Medicine State Service of the Republic of Belarus. He received his medical degree from Belarusian State Medical University, and a Master's degree in Bioethics from Union Graduate College, USA. Andrei Famenka teaches Health Law at Belarusian State Medical University and Research Ethics at the Advanced Certificate Programme in Research Ethics for Central and Eastern Europe. He is a member of the National Bioethics Committee of the Republic of Belarus. Current research interests include the ethics of international health research, social justice in healthcare and the impact of post-communist transition on the development of research ethics and clinical ethics in the countries of Central and Eastern Europe.

Kirstin Fragemann is a Professional Educator, serving as a Lecturer in Inter-professional Pain Management at the Center for Education at the University Hospital of Regensburg, Germany, since 2008. Additionally, she holds a senior staff position for Nursing Science and Quality Improvement at the Department of Nursing at the University Hospital of Regensburg, Germany. She is a Registered Nurse with clinical experience in Oncology. In 2006, she graduated from her studies in education at the University of Bremen, Germany, and focused on Nursing Science with a German University Diploma. She has established an Interprofessional Pain Education Programme at Regensburg and is co-leader of the course programme. During her career she has developed various education programmes in the fields of Pain Management. Her research focuses on interprofessional education in the context of Pain Management.

Katharina Furholzer trained as a State-Qualified Translator for Spanish before studying Scandinavian Studies, Literary Theory and Comparative Literature, and American Literary History in Munich and London. Since 2013 she has been a PhD Student at the Graduate School Practices of Literature (Münster) working on a Medical Humanities project concerned with bioethical aspects of medical and literary pathographies. Her academic work includes research assistance and teaching at the Institute for Medical History and Ethics (Halle-Wittenberg). Her research focuses on the correlations of literature, medicine and ethics, especially different forms of written medical communication as well as aspects of autonomy, coping competence and vulnerability within literature.

Sarah Galbraith joined the Palliative Care Service at Cambridge University Hospitals in 1998 while, simultaneously, working as a GP Principal in Cambridge. She was appointed as Consultant in Palliative Medicine at Cambridge University Hospitals in December 2010. Sarah's clinical work involves holistic palliative care management for patients with both malignant and non-malignant disease. She works as part of the Palliative Care Service, in a team of Doctors, Clinical Nurse Specialists, Psychologists, Occupational Therapists, Physiotherapists and Administrative Staff. Sarah's particular interest is in decision-making and ethical issues around the provision of artificial feeding for patients nearing the end of their life. Working with Gastroenterologists, Geriatricians, Speech and Language Therapists, Nutrition and Dietetic colleagues, Sarah has chaired the Feeding Issues Multidisciplinary Team weekly meeting since 2006. She is the Palliative Care lead with the Hepato-Biliary MDT. Her other research interest is the management of intractable breathlessness. Sarah has published research on the non-pharmacological management of breathlessness including the use of a handheld fan. As a result of her background in General Practice Sarah also has a particular interest in working across the interface between primary and secondary care and works closely with the CCG End of Life Board to coordinate care for patients.

Alona Goroshko is an HIV/AIDS Consultant for the World Bank Human Development Programme in Ukraine. Mrs Goroshko holds a Master's degree in Sociology and before joining the World Bank in 2013 she had been working in the area of sociological research for five years. Her professional interests include healthcare system governance, monitoring and evaluation in the health sector and social determinants of health.

Katja Götz is a Sociologist and the Deputy Head of the Department of General Practice and Health Services Research, University Hospital of Heidelberg,

Germany. Since 2008 she has held a research position at the Department of General Practice and Health Services Research at Heidelberg. In 2013, she completed her postdoctoral thesis (habilitation) in Health Services Research on the subject of the 'Working conditions of health care professionals and the impact on quality of care'. Since 2014, she has been the chairperson of Stiftung Praxissiegel e.V. Her main research interest is in quality of care, working conditions of healthcare professionals and communication between healthcare professionals and patients. She has extensive experience in qualitative and quantitative research. In addition, she has experience tutoring and supervising undergraduate, Master's, and PhD students.

Bernhard M. Graf has been Professor and Chairman of the Clinics of Anesthesiology, Intensive Care Medicine and the Air Ambulance of the University Hospital of Regensburg, Germany, since 2008. Additionally, since 2013, he has been the Vice Director of the Medical Hospital of the University of Regensburg. He has worked at various university hospitals in Germany, for example Heidelberg and Göttingen, and the United States (Children's Hospital of Wisconsin, Milwaukee). In 2006, he completed a Master of Science in Health Care Management. He has received multiple honours and awards for his research and academic teaching. During his career he has established direct simulation laboratories at Heidelberg, Göttingen and Regensburg. His special research interests focus on effects of anaesthetics, especially of pure optical isomers on different organ systems, the elderly patient in anaesthesia and on artificial organ treatment in the Intensive Care Unit.

Anthony Holland trained in Medicine at University College and University College Hospital, London, qualifying in 1973. After some years in General Medicine he then trained in Psychiatry at the Maudsley Hospital and Institute of Psychiatry in London. He held a senior academic post at the Institute of Psychiatry from 1987. In 1992 he moved to the Department of Psychiatry at the University of Cambridge and in 2002 he was appointed to the Health Foundation Chair in Learning Disability at the University of Cambridge. He leads the Cambridge Intellectual and Developmental Disabilities Research Group (www.CIDDRG.org.uk) in the Department of Psychiatry, University of Cambridge. This is a multidisciplinary group that undertakes a broad range of research relevant to people with intellectual disabilities. In 2010 he was elected a Fellow of the Academy of Medical Sciences and appointed a Senior Investigator by NIHR. For ten years until 2013 he was editor of the *Journal of Intellectual Disability Research* (JIDR). With colleagues he has undertaken studies relating to the Mental Capacity Act 2005 and was one of two advisors to the Joint Houses of Parliament Pre-legislative Scrutiny Committee examining the then Mental Incapacity Bill.

Ana Jakopec was born in 1986 in Osijek. She received a Master's degree in Psychology in 2009, defending the thesis named 'Organisational innovation diagnosis: a case study at the University of Osijek'. She was awarded a PhD in Psychology in 2015 at the University of Rijeka, defending the dissertation entitled 'Effects of (mis)alignment between organisational, supervisory and peer justice climate'. In 2010, she started working as a Teaching Assistant at the Department of Psychology, Faculty of Humanities and Social Sciences, University of Osijek. Before this she spent a year and a half working as a Professional Associate-Psychologist in the Electrical Engineering and Traffic School in Osijek. Her occupational field is Work and Organisational Psychology. She is a collaborator on the scientific project 'Determinants and effects of the organisational (in)justice', funded by the University of Rijeka. Also, within the EFPSA Junior Researcher Programme, she is leading an international team of six young researchers in the research project on the topic of 'Work engagement and performance'. She has published 12 scientific papers and presented the results of her research at 19 international and national conferences. She is a member of the Croatian Psychological Association, Croatian Psychological Chamber and European Association of Work and Organisational Psychology.

Nicole Lindenberg is a Psychotherapist in cognitive-behavioural therapy. Since 2006, she has been working in the Department of Pain Medicine, which is part of the Clinics of Anaesthesiology and Intensive Care Medicine of the University Hospital of Regensburg, Germany. She graduated her studies in Psychology at the University of Regensburg, focused on Clinical Psychology and Family Psychology with a German University Diploma and completed university training as a Pain Expert. Since 2009, she has been a Lecturer in Pain Management. She is doing research into attitude to pain in Pain Therapists.

Cornelia Mahler is a Registered Nurse and Programme Coordinator of the Bachelor of Science – Interprofessional Health Care at the Medical Faculty, University of Heidelberg. She is Vice Chairperson of the Working Group on Interprofessional Education for the German Medical Education Association. Since 2005, she has held a research position at the Department of General Practice and Health Services Research, University Hospital Heidelberg. In 2010, she completed her doctoral thesis in Health Services Research on the subject of 'Medication communication in general practice: instrument development and evaluation from a patient perspective'. She also holds a Master of Educational Science from the University of Heidelberg, Germany. Her research is focused on the evaluation and measurement of interprofessional education and interprofessional collaboration. Other research interests include nursing assessments, complementary nursing, medication management and coordination of care.

Alex McKeown is a Postdoctoral Teaching Associate in Bioethics at the University of Bristol Centre for Ethics in Medicine, where he studied for his PhD and held a Postdoctoral Research Associate position. Previously Alex was a Postdoctoral Researcher in Public Health at the University of East London Institute for Health and Human Development. Prior to this, Alex spent three years working in genetics education research for the charity Genetic Alliance UK. He coordinated a project funded by the European Commission for Life Sciences and Biotechnology which aimed to improve information for patients and health professionals about informed consent and biobanking in genetic testing and research across Europe. Before this, he took a BA in Philosophy and an MA in Healthcare Ethics at the University of Leeds. Alex's primary orientation is philosophical, although he is interested in interdisciplinary research. In his PhD he carried out some empirical work, the data from which informed the philosophical analysis. Currently, Alex's primary research interest is the intersection between human enhancement and public health. This follows from his PhD, and the research which enabled his contribution here was funded by a Wellcome Trust Society and Ethics Small Grant project entitled 'Ethics, Enhancement, and Public Health'.

Christopher Philbey is a specialist in Endocrinology from the United Kingdom with a background in Medical Anthropology. He is Chief Operating Officer of two charities associated with healthcare and ethical resource usage. Between these two commitments, he is also active in the field of ecological and wildlife conservation, regularly travelling across the globe to volunteer with wildlife sanctuaries and habitat protection agencies.

Stephanie Rüsch is Research Associate at the Faculty of Business, Economics and Social Science at TU Dortmund University in Germany. After obtaining her Master's degree in Economic Sciences in 2013, she started her PhD project in the field of management and accounting in the healthcare sector. Her research focuses on strategic management, performance measurement and management control. Her contributions have been accepted at renowned conferences such as the European Academy of Management and the European Group for Organizational Studies.

Sabine Salloch graduated in Medicine and Philosophy from the University of Marburg and has two years' working experience as a Physician in Internal Medicine. She is working as a Researcher at the Institute for Medical Ethics and History of Medicine, Ruhr-University Bochum, Germany. Her research interests are in Clinical Ethics (decision-making in oncology, ethical issues at the end of life), Medical Professionalism (ethics and economy, interprofessional teaching) and the methodology of empirical–ethical research. She recently finished her PhD dissertation which deals with the subject of practical judgement ('*Urteilskraft*') in Applied Ethics. Her work has been awarded with scholarships and prizes, for example by the Ethox Centre (University of Oxford), the Akademie für Ethik in der Medizin (AEM) and The North Rhine-Westphalian Academy of Sciences, Humanities and the Arts.

Verena Sandow is a freelance Project Manager and Coordinator. She is a trained Philosopher and scientist in the field of Medical Ethics and Applied Ethics. Following her studies in Philosophy, Media Studies and Economic History at the Heinrich-Heine-University Düsseldorf, she was a member of the research training group 'Bioethics' at the International Centre in Science and Humanities, Eberhard-Karls-University, Tübingen. She worked in the fields of Human Medical Research and Research Ethics and co-organised several conferences in the field of Medical Ethics at the Institute for Medical Ethics and History of Medicine, Ruhr-University Bochum, Germany.

Jan Schildmann studied Medicine at the Charité Medical School, Berlin, and received an MA in Medical Law and Ethics from King's College, University of London. He has qualified as a specialist in Internal Medicine and is a Senior Researcher at the Institute of Medical Ethics and History of Medicine, Ruhr-University Bochum, Germany. His research covers various topics in Clinical Ethics (e.g. ethics in Oncology and Palliative Care, ethics support services) and methodological aspects of combining normative and empirical analysis in Medical Ethics. In addition he has developed teaching modules on professional aspects of medicine (e.g. breaking bad news, interprofessional collaboration and risk communication) for students and healthcare professionals. His work has been published in a broad range of ethics and medical journals and awarded with several research prizes.

Jobst-Hendrik Schultz is a Senior Physician at the Department of General Internal Medicine and Psychosomatics and Head of Medical Education at the Department of Internal Medicine, University Hospital Heidelberg, Germany. He started his research career in the Department of Physiology. In 2010, he completed his postdoctoral thesis (habilitation) in Physiology on the subject of the 'Molecular characteristics of single isolated cardio-myocytes'. Since 2012, he has been Head of Psychocardiology at the Department of General Internal Medicine and Psychosomatics, University Hospital Heidelberg. His main clinical research interest is in comorbidity of depression and heart failure. He has extensive experience in qualitative and quantitative research on doctor–patient communication and also assessment in medical education.

Martina Šendula-Pavelić is a graduate Psychologist, born in 1973 in Rijeka. Since 1997, she has worked as a Professional Associate-Psychologist in high schools, counselling and teaching different courses and leading psychology workshops (Work and Marketing Psychology, Management Skills, Culture of Communicating and others), as well as being a Senior Advisor for professional guidance and education in the Croatian Employment Service. Since 2011, she has been working as a Lecturer at the Department of Social Sciences and Medical Humanities, Faculty of Medicine and at the Public Health Department, Faculty of Health Studies at University of Rijeka, teaching Medical Ethics, Scientific Methodology and Communication Skills.

She is a collaborator on the scientific project 'Determinants and effects of the organisational (in)justice', funded by the University of Rijeka. In 2013, she enrolled in a postgraduate (doctoral) university study programme in Biomedicine at the Medical Faculty in Rijeka. She is a member of the Croatian Bioethics Society, Croatian Society for Clinical Bioethics, Croatian Psychological Chamber and Croatian Psychological Association. She is interested in the psychology and neuroscience of morality, as well as in improving the quality of education and methodology of teaching. Her current work focuses on investigating ethical leadership in healthcare settings, its consequences and the ways for empowering ethical competence and ethical climate in the workplace.

Dorina Maria Stănescu's interests are in Applied Ethics, Normative Ethics, Global Justice and Political Philosophy. She holds a PhD in Philosophy from Universitad Autonoma de Barcelona, where she defended the thesis 'A moral investigation of the brain drain of healthcare professionals: The Rawls–Nozick debate framework'. Between 2005 and 2008 she attended courses in Moral and Political Philosophy at the Faculty of Philosophy, University of Bucharest. Between 2008 and 2010 she attended the Master's course in Applied Ethics at the Faculty of Philosophy, University of Bucharest with an Erasmus scholarship at University Autonoma de Barcelona.

Tetiana Stepurko is Assistant Professor and Head of Master Programme 'Health care management' at the School of Public Health, National University of Kyiv–Mohyla Academy. She is a member of the organisational committee for the 'Health care system transformation: Eastern Europe' Summer School. In 2013 she obtained her PhD degree from Maastricht University, the Netherlands, with research focused on the nature and scale of informal patient payments in Central and Eastern European countries. Apart from informal payments in healthcare, her research interests include organisation of healthcare service provision as well as its gender and social structure aspects.

Zoran Sušanj was born in 1962 in Rijeka. He graduated in Psychology at the University of Rijeka, obtained an MA in Psychology at the University of Ljubljana, and a PhD in Psychology at the University of Zagreb. First, he served as a Psychologist in the Personnel Department of a petrochemical company DINA, Omišalj. From 1986, he has worked at the Department of Psychology, Faculty of Humanities and Social Sciences, University of Rijeka, and currently he is an Associate Professor lecturing in Organisational Psychology, Psychology of Leadership and Organisational Development. During 1992, he served as a Military Psychologist in the Croatian Army. From 1997, he worked as a Management Consultant, mostly on projects of strategic planning and management, leadership training, and implementing organisational changes through the improvement of human resources function in various organisations. He has published about 40 scientific and professional papers and two books in the field of Work and Organisational Psychology. He has participated in and led different domestic and international scientific projects researching work motivation, leadership, organisational climate and culture. Currently he leads the scientific project 'Determinants and effects of the organisational (in)justice', funded by the University of Rijeka. He is a member of the Croatian Psychological Association, Croatian Psychological Chamber and European Association of Work and Organisational Psychology.

Joachim Szecsenyi is a Family Physician and Sociologist. He is Professor and Head of the Department of General Practice and Health Services Research and also Director and Co-Founder of the Institute for Applied Quality Improvement and Research in Health Care (AQUA-Institute) in Göttingen – a large independent and impartial corporation that provides services for healthcare quality assurance in the German health system. He has more than 25 years' working experience in quality improvement research and health services research. From 2001 to 2007 he was president of the European Association for Quality in Family Practice (EQuiP), an organisation that collaborates intensively with developing countries. Professor Szecsenyi has written more than 300 scientific publications on these issues. Since 2009 he has been head of the nationwide system of hospital benchmarking and transsectoral quality of care in Germany, funded by the Federal Joint Committee 'Gemeinsamer Bundesausschuss'.

Clemens Tangerding has studied at the universities of Münster and Würzburg and received his PhD at the Technical University of Dresden and the École Pratique des Hautes Études in Paris. In his thesis, he analysed the influence of the political changes of the Napoleonic Era on five specific professions. He has published numerous works on the history of Protestant hospitals. He delivers lectures at the University of Gießen and the Free University Berlin.

Jochen Vollmann is a Physician and Medical Ethicist. He serves as Professor and Director of the Institute for Medical Ethics and History of Medicine and President of the Centre for Medical Ethics, Ruhr-University Bochum, Germany. Professor Vollmann was Visiting Fellow at the Kennedy Institute of Ethics, Georgetown University, Washington DC, Visiting Professor at the San Francisco School of Medicine, New York, at the Institute for the Medical Humanities UTMB, Texas and at the Centre for Values, Ethics and the Law in Medicine at the University of Sydney. He was honoured with the Prize for Brain Research in Geriatrics of the University of Witten/ Herdecke, the Stehr-Boldt-Prize for Medical Ethics of the University of Zurich, the Research Award of the German Association of Palliative Medicine, as well as the University Teaching Award 'lehrreich' of the Ruhr-University Bochum and the 'Gaudium docendi' Teaching Award of the Society of Friends and Sponsors of the Ruhr-University Bochum.

Professor Vollmann's research interests include informed consent and capacity assessment, mental health ethics, end-of-life decision-making, advance directives, personalised medicine, medical professionalism, clinical ethics committees and clinical ethics consultation.

Christoph H. R. Wiese is Senior Physician and Chief of the Department of Pain Medicine, which is part of the Clinics of Anaesthesiology and Intensive Care Medicine of the University Hospital of Regensburg, Germany. He completed his Anaesthesia residency training at the University of Göttingen, Germany, in 2004. Additionally he holds certifications by the German Medical Association in Pain Medicine, Palliative Care, Intensive Care Medicine and Emergency Medicine. He has extensive training and experience in the treatment of acute and chronic pain conditions, including cancer pain. Christoph Wiese is an active author and educator in the field of Pain Medicine, Palliative Care and Emergency Medicine. He has established an interprofessional pain education programme at Regensburg and is co-leader of the course programme. He has received multiple awards and honours for his research. During his career he has developed various education programmes in the fields of Pain Management. In 2012 he obtained his Master of Health Business Administration at the University of Nuremberg/Erlangen, Germany.

Jeremy Woodward is a Consultant Gastroenterologist at Addenbrooke's Hospital where he runs the service for intestinal failure and artificial nutrition and is one of the lead physicians in the national intestinal and multivisceral transplant service. He was instrumental in establishing the Feeding Issues multidisciplinary team with colleagues in 2006 and places the majority of the enteral feeding tubes in the Trust. He has published original research in intestinal failure, coeliac disease and nutrition and has a particular interest in nutrition support at the end of life.

Tim Wray is a recent graduate of Medicine from the University of East Anglia with prior interest and academic study at the University of Southampton in the fields of Biomedical Sciences, Pharmacology and Proteomics.

Christopher Yu is a Hospital Physician currently working in Northern England. He graduated from the University of Sheffield Medical School in 2013 with a specialist interest in Anaesthetics and Intensive Care Medicine. Alongside this he has an interest in the effects of hierarchy on teams within the workplace.

1 Introduction

Sabine Salloch, Verena Sandow,
Jan Schildmann and Jochen Vollmann

Ethics and professionalism in healthcare – a brief introduction

Physicians served for a long time as a paradigm example of an occupation that is distinguished by certain features which transform it from a 'mere job' into a *profession*. Members of a profession bear specific characteristics, such as a specialised academic education, working autonomy, professional bodies, self-government and codes of ethics (Carr-Saunders and Wilson, 1933; Dingwall, 1983; Freidson, 2001). Medical doctors, as highly qualified academics whose work is very much shaped by complex regulatory and organisational structures, can be regarded as indicative of the chances and challenges which are associated with professionalism in modern societies. Some of the key features of professionalism are closely linked to the basic principles of medical ethics, such as autonomy, beneficence and justice (Beauchamp and Childress, 2013), while other aspects (such as the establishment of a professional association or high compensation) do not refer directly to morally demanded tasks.

The notion of professionalism within medicine and healthcare has recently gained attention as a countermovement to forces and tendencies which threaten the independent judgement of physicians regarding the care of individual patients and for the sake of society (ABIM Foundation, 2002). Along these lines, a renewed sense of professionalism supports the efforts to ensure that healthcare professionals and healthcare systems remain committed to patient welfare and the basic tenets of social justice. Furthermore, professional judgement and behaviour have increasingly become part of undergraduate medical curricula (General Medical Council, 2005; CanMEDS, 2015; NKLM, 2015) and even play a role in the distribution of job opportunities in some countries. Professionalism is, thus, currently high on the agenda of medical education, healthcare providers and key players in the international reform of healthcare systems.

Despite this general tendency, the theoretical underpinnings of healthcare professionalism and its manifold appearance in everyday practice remain widely unexplored. In addition to the traditional profession of the medical doctor, a large number of other healthcare vocations have appeared on the scene and passed enormous processes of professionalisation during the last few decades. The spectrum of professionals has widened enormously from the beginning of professional nursing in the nineteenth century up to the development of more and more specialised assisting vocations, such as orthoptist or speech and language therapists. There are also considerable international differences in the training, role and status of non-physician healthcare professionals. While many countries have already established academic training for nurses and assisting vocations, there are other countries, such as Germany, in which the division between academic training for physicians and an apprenticeship for other healthcare staff still prevails (Friedrichs and Schaub, 2011).

This volume presents the results of an interdisciplinary conference on ethics and professionalism in healthcare which was organised by the Institute for Medical Ethics and History of Medicine at Ruhr-University Bochum, Germany. The conference took place in Bochum from 9 to 13 February 2015 and was funded by the German Federal Ministry of Education and Research (BMBF; 01GP1387). The topic of ethics and professionalism in healthcare attracted considerable attention and the organisers received the high number of 83 applications, which far exceeded the number of funded places available. Therefore, a selection was made of contributions which, on the one hand, promised innovative ideas on the topic of professionalism in healthcare and, on the other hand, included researchers from a wide range of countries (Belarus, Croatia, Germany, Great Britain, Romania and Ukraine), as well as participants with a more theoretical and practice-oriented approach to the topic. The outcome of this competitive selection process was a programme that sheds light onto various aspects of ethics and professionalism in healthcare from both international and multi-professional perspectives.

This book summarises the conference results and is structured into five main parts. Each chapter has undergone significant revisions following the conference and has gone through an extensive peer review process. The book concludes with a joint position paper which brings together the junior scientists' main ideas on the status quo of, and future perspectives for, healthcare professionalism. The following paragraphs will provide an overview of the book's content.

Part I – Historical and societal aspects of healthcare professions

In order to better understand the shifting requirements and dynamic roles of professionals in modern healthcare, a look at their historical development and social context is of great importance. The perspectives of history and medical humanities can help to set current questions into a new context and illuminate aspects that would have otherwise slipped the attention of the researcher. Consequently, the two contributions in the first part of the book highlight aspects of healthcare professionalism that are not often in the focus of modern discussions, but nevertheless, sharpen our view of the role of professionals in the clinical context.

Clemens Tangerding examines the role of religious institutions as hospital owners in his historical analysis. He focuses on the period of transition between the 1960s and the 1980s, in which many of these institutions handed over nursing care and clinic management to secular agencies. Tangerding shows how the first generation of secular nurses strongly advocated political awareness and a strengthening of their working rights, which led to increased employee representation. The author characterises these developments as 'a shifting focus from patients to employees' and discusses how far nursing in the twenty-first century can only be successful when it is still regarded as a profession.

The focus of the second contribution, by Katharina Fürholzer, is on physician–patient communication. She expands the oral doctor–patient communication on a written level by analysing the possible effects of the author–reader relationship on the doctor–patient relationship. Physician's letters, as a particular type of text, still lack systematic research and teaching, which can turn into an ethically relevant problem when the patient becomes the actual but unintended reader of their own pathography. Fürholzer argues that it is time to raise awareness of the possible correlations between written and spoken doctor–patient interactions, which are equally vital for today's understanding of medical professionalism.

Part II – Learning and teaching healthcare professionalism

The dynamic interactions between the various healthcare vocations necessitate a better reflection on the learning and teaching of healthcare professionalism. Healthcare teams must function collaboratively and optimally utilise all the different competencies available for the care of individual patients. This brings about the need for new standards in the education of physicians and non-physician healthcare professionals. Issues of interprofessional collaboration are increasingly integrated in the respective curricula.

Sarah Berger *et al.* provide an overview of existing models, such as shared decision-making, and propose a collaborative decision-making model for use in interprofessional healthcare teams. Collaborative decision-making is seen as a complex phenomenon which aims at reaching decisions amenable to all stakeholders, even in the event of varying objectives or conflicting interests. The authors highlight that equipping healthcare professionals to work together effectively is an important means to optimise patient care outcomes in complex healthcare environments.

Kirstin Fragemann *et al.* take up the example of pain management and introduce an integrated interprofessional pain curriculum for healthcare professionals ('Pain Care Manager'). This postgraduate programme was designed by a six-step approach to curriculum development for clinically experienced healthcare staff, such as physicians, nurses, psychologists, physiotherapists, occupational health therapists and pharmacists. The programme evaluation suggests the acceptance of interprofessional learning approaches and encourages further activities in the field of ongoing education.

Part III – Transformation of healthcare professions

Professional roles and expectations concerning healthcare professionals have undergone a significant change in the last few years due to societal and political developments. Post-Soviet countries in particular are currently experiencing a situation of instability which affects the working conditions of physicians heavily. In addition to that, the problem of the international 'brain drain' poses severe challenges to Eastern European healthcare systems.

Tetiana Stepurko *et al.*, in their qualitative empirical study, analyse recent approaches of assuring professionalism among medical staff in the Ukraine. They identify a range of problems in the area of internal governance which affect physicians' professionalism. According to their findings, professional development is perceived mostly as the personal responsibility of the physician. This poses multiple-nature barriers to the enforcement of healthcare professionalism and, therefore, challenges the adequate access to and quality of healthcare services in the Ukraine.

Andrei Famenka provides an overview of the situation of Clinical Ethics Consultation (CEC) in Belarus and analyses how it functions on the basis of a modified framework by Hyder *et al.* (2009). The current regulation of Healthcare Ethics Committees in Belarus is centralised and strict. Famenka argues that a number of factors of socio-political and economic post-communist transition in Belarus are responsible for creating an environment in which the operations of CEC services are adversarial to ethical reflection and democratisation. The notion of professionalism is used as a means to exercise control over the medical profession for the sake of certain societal and political interests.

Dorina Maria Stănescu discusses the right of healthcare professionals to free movement and emigration from their country of origin in her contribution on the international brain drain. Stănescu embraces Nozick's libertarian view that we owe others no more than that which the term of a formal contract signed in total agreement requires. She concludes that healthcare professionals have no moral duty to stay in their country of birth and education because they are not bound by any agreement with the citizens of their country of origin and that they have no moral duty to fix their respective healthcare systems.

Part IV – Professional leadership and team decision-making in healthcare

Contemporary healthcare professionalism is executed in multidisciplinary teams. Therefore, team structures and leadership play a key role in ensuring high-quality patient care. Issues of professional leadership and team decision-making are discussed by three case studies from the UK, Croatia and Germany, respectively.

Gemma Clarke *et al.* report on a qualitative observational study on multi-professional team meetings concerning feeding interventions for patients at risk of lacking capacity. The authors found that the decisions concerning artificial nutrition and hydration are complex and multifaceted. The decision-making is not a one-off choice, but involves many different steps and decisions and includes discussions with relatives and other clinicians taking place both before and after the team meetings. The study further reveals that decisions in clinical practice may contain elements of both substituted and supported decision-making.

Regarding their questionnaire study, Martina Šendula-Pavelić *et al.* start from the idea of ethical leaders as role models, whose integrity, honesty and fair treatment encourage ethical behaviour within the organisation. The research was conducted on a convenience sample of Croatian healthcare teams and examined the relationship between healthcare team members' perceptions of the ethical leadership of their supervisors and the team members' own attitudes and behaviours. As a result, ethical leadership was positively related to all the desirable attitudinal, motivational and behavioural outcomes of the team members.

Management as a 'third profession' in healthcare is the subject of a qualitative interview study by Stephanie Rüsch. She analyses the cooperation between hospital managers and physicians in the context of strategy-making processes. Her findings reveal that chief physicians are considerably involved in strategic decision-making, while, at the same time, managers are gaining increasing control over medical services. Rüsch concludes that the traditional image of professional bureaucracy should be critically discussed and she provides suggestions regarding altered organisational structures within hospitals.

Part V – Ethical challenges to healthcare professionalism

The classic notion of medical professionalism refers to the idea of the individual physician making treatment decisions based on the best available scientific evidence and for the sake of his patients. However, in clinical reality, this image gets shaken by organisational and hierarchical structures and societal developments which counteract the ideal picture of professional autonomy. Becoming and acting as a medical professional means more than exercising knowledge and competencies based on formal training. The two last contributions in this volume highlight the complex socialisation of junior doctors and the increasing importance of physicians in the context of public health.

Tim Wray *et al.* analyse the phenomenon of akrasia in situations where junior doctors, despite their belief, still carry out a senior's strategy against their own moral conscience. Starting from a clinical case example, the authors discuss psychological studies on conformity and obedience and link it to the workplace reality in hospitals. They come to the conclusion that a lack of senior support causes moral stress in the early training of physicians and that constructive feedback and flatter hierarchies can help to address this.

In the last chapter, Alex McKeown highlights the increasing importance of prevention in modern medicine. As healthcare provision should respond to the needs of society, medical professionals have to rethink the boundaries of their work. McKeown especially discusses the role of biomedical enhancement from a public health perspective and stresses that a growing commitment to the optimisation of healthy longevity has consequences for the notion of healthcare professionalism.

The editors thank all the authors for their chapters and their willingness to contribute to the volume. We also thank the German Federal Ministry of Education and Research (BMBF) for its financial support without which the overall project and this book would not have been possible. Finally, we are thankful to Philip Saunders for proofreading and formatting the manuscripts and to Routledge for their longstanding professional cooperation.

References

ABIM Foundation, 2002. Medical professionalism in the new millennium: a physician charter. *Annals of Internal Medicine*, 136(3), pp. 243–6.
Beauchamp, T.L. and Childress, J.F., 2013. *Principles of Biomedical Ethics*. 7th Ed. Oxford: Oxford University Press.
CanMEDS Physician Competency Framework 2015. Available through: <www.royalcollege.ca/portal/page/portal/rc/common/documents/canmeds/framework/canmeds2015_framework_series_IV_e.pdf> [accessed 5 August 2015].
Carr-Saunders, A. and Wilson, P.A., 1933. *The Professions*. Oxford: Oxford University Press.
Dingwall, R. ed., 1983. *The Sociology of the Professions. Lawyers, doctors and others*. London: Macmillan.
Freidson, E., 2001. *Professionalism. The third logic*. Cambridge: Polity.
Friedrichs, A. and Schaub, H.-A., 2011. Academisation of the health professions – achievements and future prospects. *GMS Z Med Ausbild*, 28(4), p. doc50.
General Medical Council, 2005. Medical students: professional values and fitness to practise. Available through: <awww.gmc-uk.org/education/undergraduate/professional_behaviour.asp> [accessed 5 August 2015].
Hyder, A.A., Dawson, L., Bachani, A.M. and Lavery, J., 2009. Moving from research ethics review to research ethics systems in low-income and middle-income countries. *Lancet*, 373, pp. 862–5.
NKLM: Nationaler Kompetenzbasierter Lernzielkatalog Medizin, 2015. Kapitel 11 Die Ärztin und der Arzt als professionell Handelnde/-r. Available through: <www.nklm.de/kataloge/nklm/lernziel/uebersicht> [accessed 5 August 2015].

Part I

Historical and societal aspects of healthcare professions

2 A shifting focus from patients to employees

Withdrawal of religious communities
and the emergence of political activity
in Protestant hospitals in Berlin
between 1960 and 1990

Clemens Tangerding

German Protestant hospitals were subject to two major transformations between 1960 and 1990. Protestant hospitals here are defined as hospitals belonging to the Diakonia, which is the social welfare branch of the Protestant Church in Germany. The term Protestant here is the translation of the German term *evangelisch*. I use it in the same sense as McLeod (1982, p. 323) and Zerull (2011, p. 89). On the one hand, the motherhouses were in the last stages of withdrawing from hospital care and management; the sisterhoods ceased their involvement in the wards. On the other hand, the trade unions were increasingly gaining power. While the withdrawal of the sisterhoods brought an end to a longstanding tradition, the entry of the unions marked the beginning of a historical development with consequences lasting until today. As these two significant processes happened at the same time, the entire representation of the hospital changed. Until then, the public had thought of hospitals as places where patients were healed and cared for. They now became centres of trade union activity and sites of conflict between management and employees, in other words, a political space. The focus both inside and outside the hospitals shifted rather unconsciously from patients to caregivers and doctors.

This chapter begins by introducing the sources used for research and by setting the methodological framework. In the second part, the situation up until the 1970s is illustrated. The third part addresses the withdrawal process as it took place in the four specific hospitals to which this contribution refers. The fourth part examines the appearance of politically active employees among caregivers and doctors. The fifth and final part sums up these observations and draws some conclusions on how the withdrawal of the sisterhoods affected the general public's perception of hospitals.

Sources and methods

The main source used for this chapter are board meeting minutes from the Association for the Foundation of Protestant Hospitals (*Verein zur Errichtung evangelischer Krankenhäuser*). This organisation, which belonged to the Diakonia, was founded in 1928 and it owned three and operated one of the four hospitals analysed below. The association changed its name into the *Paul Gerhardt Diakonie* in 2009, and owns all of the four hospitals in Berlin today. The minutes have never been used for historical research before. Most of the files are written minutes and not just summaries. Additionally, they contain writings and documents with which the board members dealt in their professional daily routines, as well as parts of correspondence between the chairman of the board and other officeholders, for example, superiors of motherhouses. The author of this contribution has written monographs on all four hospitals, therefore, in most cases, these publications will be quoted rather than the original sources, because the former are more accessible. Besides using the minutes as a main resource, this chapter also draws on publications by the Association for the Foundation of Protestant Hospitals. Those were published mainly in order to attract new supporters and raise money. Other sources include correspondence between clinic managers and medical directors or the superiors of the motherhouses and sisterhoods involved. Although each motherhouse consisted of sisterhoods, it seems necessary here to differentiate between relatively strict motherhouses and the more liberal Protestant sisterhoods, which allowed their member nurses to easily quit the community on their own terms, for example, to get married.

All four hospitals are located in Berlin and belong to the Diakonia: the Protestant Elisabeth Clinic Berlin (formerly *Elisabeth-Krankenhaus des Frauen-Kranken-Vereins* and *Elisabeth-Diakonissen- und Krankenhaus*), founded in 1837, the Martin Luther Hospital Berlin and the Protestant Hubertus Hospital, both founded in 1931, and the *Evangelisches Waldkrankenhaus Spandau*, founded in 1946.

The nurses who worked in these hospitals were not all part of the same religious community. The nurses at the Elisabeth Hospital were deaconesses and belonged to the motherhouse of the same name. It was members of the Protestant Diakonia Association who were responsible for providing care at the Martin Luther Hospital and the Protestant *Waldkrankenhaus Spandau*. When the Hubertus Hospital was founded, the management concluded a contract with the Deaconess House (*Diakonissenhaus*) Lehnin in Brandenburg, which continued to staff the wards until the end of the Second World War. After the war, they returned to their home in Lehnin. Following a short transitional period, hospital management reached an agreement with the Sisterhood of the Protestant Union Dessau (*Schwesternschaft des Evangelischen Bundes in Dessau*; Tangerding, 2011a, p. 51).

As to its methodological approach, this research uses document analysis (Landwehr, 2008; Bowen, 2009, pp. 27–40) to systematically analyse the major transformation taking place in Protestant hospitals between 1970 and 1990. It draws on the two methodological traditions of content analysis (Mayring, 2000) and discourse analysis (Keller 2007, pp. 79–92; Rapley 2007), in order to provide a thorough description of the real changes within the hospitals and their context, on the one hand, and to identify changing perceptions of the relevant actors at the time, particularly members of management and staff, on the other. The aim of the study is, first, to describe the process of change in its very context, which includes outlining crucial developments at legal, administrative, organisational and labour market levels; and, second, to identify broader patterns not only in the practices of the actors involved, but also in their self-perception, which, as we will see, contributed fundamentally to turning the hospitals into a political space. Note, however, that the emphasis on analysing the use of language in this study is far weaker than in historical discourse analysis, let alone critical discourse analysis.

Protestant communities in hospitals

> Is the Lord not gracious and his kindness not invariably the same today, that he enables us in these days of misery – when everyone is moaning and lamenting – simply by way of charitable gifts to kindly care for so many sick who are abandoned, poor, often suffering and perishing miserably, and to feed them, to provide them with a doctor, medicine, and all that is needed, and to sustain and revive them for so many days. Yes, it is the purest and highest pleasure and a sacred joy to not merely be a witness but be given the opportunity to arrange for this!
>
> (Gossner, 1849, p. 3)

These words date back to the year 1848 and were probably written by Johannes Gossner, priest and head of the Association who ran the Elisabeth Hospital. The full name until 1895 was the 'Elisabeth Hospital of the Association of Sick Women' (*Elisabeth-Krankenhaus des Frauen-Kranken-Vereins*). The association was led by a priest, the hospital by a matron. These two formed the management of the hospital, which, in the beginning, was only one branch of the association (von Rotenhan, 1962, p. 56; Tangerding, 2012, pp. 7, 51). Gossner felt it was by the grace of God that the nurses were allowed to heal the sick at the Protestant hospital. Service to the sick was service to God. We find this self-concept not only in the annual reports of the sisterhood which was responsible for patient care at the Elisabeth Hospital in Berlin. What we consider a motherhouse only developed from around 1860 onwards (von Rothenhan, 1962, p. 56; Wolff and Wolff, 2002, pp. 10–36; Tangerding, 2012, p. 51) The idea of nursing as a labour of love (*Liebesdienst*; Kreutzer, 2005) was commonplace in German hospitals from the early nineteenth century onwards. Sisterhoods engaging in patient care were formed in all of the existent member states of the German Confederation.

The introduction of health insurance in the German Empire in 1883 and, to a certain extent, demographic growth raised the need for hospitals and beds. The population grew by 30 per cent in the last quarter of the nineteenth century and hospitals were needed urgently. The number of hospitals increased from 3,000 to 6,100 and beds from 141,000 to 370,000. This development was due primarily to the introduction of health insurance, although insurance was only mandatory for a small number of people in the beginning, and decades went by until the majority of workers and employees were covered (Möller and Hesselbarth, 1998, p. 97; Kaufmann, 2003, p. 270).

This process strengthened the motherhouse system. In fact, the involvement of religious communities in hospital care in the nineteenth and twentieth centuries was quite diversified. Seidler and Leven (2003) have identified four different providers of hospital care in the nineteenth century: Catholic orders, secular associations of motherhouses, non-affiliated nurses (Seidler and Leven, 2003, p. 209) and the Protestant Diakonia. Non-affiliated nurses did not play a very important role in hospital care at the national level until the end of the Second World War, although there was remarkable progress between 1900 and 1933 with regard to their level of organisation, especially in the big cities. The situation was different in home care (*Privatpflege*), because independent nurses had started to play a crucial role here since the last quarter of the nineteenth century (Seidler and Leven, 2003, p. 223). Regarding the other three groups, communities differed remarkably as to size, prevalence and continuity. Most motherhouses of the Protestant Diakonia originated from Kaiserswerth, near Düsseldorf, but were only loosely connected to their founding centre and conducted largely independent operations. Things were also inconsistent on the Catholic side. There was a wide spectrum ranging from tiny communities, focusing only on specific regions, for example, the Catherine sisters, to branches of large orders, such as the Sisters of Charity (Wolff and Wolff, 2002, p. 10; Seidler and Leven, 2003, p. 210). Women's communities were responsible for patient care and administration in the vast majority of cases, but there were a few exceptions of Catholic men's orders, such as the Alexian Brothers, with headquarters in Münster (Bildstein, Groß and Kühl, 2009, pp. 39–56). Despite this patchwork situation of how hospital care was organised, it appears that the motherhouse system also dominated Catholic caregiving. This is also true for the secular branches of motherhouses. There were nursing communities with a strong anti-ecclesiastical claim and a Protestant tinge, such as the Victoria Sisters. This organisation was cofounded by the Berlin-based pathologist and public health politician Rudolf Virchow. For Virchow, it was very important to draw a clear line between the ecclesiastical motherhouses and the Victoria Sisters. Virchow (1869) gave a famous talk at a Berlin conference in which he outlined the sisterhood's anti-ecclesiastical approach. Nevertheless, the everyday environment in this community did not differ much from the daily lives of deaconesses and nuns. The community members preferably lived together, comparable to a motherhouse; they were led by a matron or superior and could be sent out to establish new communities; and they were bound by instructions and not paid directly by the hospital but by their community. No work contract usually existed between the nurses and hospital management. The Victoria Sisters were sent to the wards of the city-owned hospitals, such as Friedrichshain and Urban Hospital. The community was founded in 1881 and dissolved in 1920 when the sisters became public servants. A study on the Victoria Sisters does not yet exist (Wolff and Wolff, 1994, p. 156; Seidler and Leven, 2003, p. 225; see also Bolk,

1984, p. 59; Schweikardt, 2004, p. 209). In a way, the motherhouses mono-
polised sick care in hospitals until the end of the Second World War. Not
least the National Socialist Sisterhood blended national socialist ideology
with the organisational and hierarchical structure of a motherhouse (Breiding,
1998, p. 87).

The term monopoly does not apply to the theological foundations of nursing within the religious communities. The theological legacy of self-sacrifice
within the nursing profession was closely linked with religious denomination.
Worshipping saints was part of everyday prayers in Catholic hospitals, whereas
Protestant-led ones regarded not only the veneration in itself, but also the
founding of Catholic hospitals named after saints with scepticism. The hospital
of St Joseph, for example, was founded in 1928 and the hospital of St Hildegard
in 1926. Confessional rivalry in general, the antagonism between Protestant
deaconess motherhouses and Catholic orders, as well as competition between
hospitals owned by political communities and those managed by religious
organisations, played an important role in how the sisterhoods defined themselves (Nipperdey, 1988; Tangerding, 2015). Motherhouses differed, above all,
with regard to the legacy of self-sacrifice for the sick. The sisters were normally
aware of the main theological ideas of the founding father or mother of
their sisterhood and often repeated them during services, prayers and in their
publications. The deaconesses of the St Elisabeth motherhouse in Berlin, for
example, regularly quoted scriptures by the founding father Johannes Gossner
in their magazine *Greetings from the Elisabeth Hospital* (*Grüße aus dem Elisabeth-
Krankenhaus*), published from 1914 to 1939. These aspects of nursing, however,
will not be dealt with in this chapter (Käppeli, 2004, p. 281).

Sisters joined a Protestant community for different reasons. A crucial one
was the aspect of being cared for. Religious communities created a safe haven
for one or more of a family's children, where they would be looked after
and could live in stable conditions (Schwarz, 1998, p. 161). Furthermore, and
importantly, women were offered the rare opportunity of learning a profession
by joining a community and training to become a nurse. This aspect applied
particularly to the Protestant motherhouse movement and far less to the
Catholic sisterhoods. Consequently, when, from about 1890 on, the opportunity was provided for women to become nurses without entering a motherhouse, the Protestant world was stirred up much more than the Catholic one
(Schwarz, 1998, p. 218). The new choices for women led to the founding of
the Diakonia Association, which offered a nurse training, but allowed its
members to leave the organisation afterwards (Schwarz, 1998, pp. 29, 234;
Seidler and Leven, 2003, p. 214).

After joining a community and training in nursing care, the women worked
– almost without interruption – by the patients' beds and in the operating
rooms. The work schedule differed from one hospital to another, but nurses
usually had only one day off and worked six days a week (Kreutzer, 2008).
A so-called split shift was common. Work started early in the morning between
five and seven a.m. and initially went on until twelve a.m. and two p.m., then

there was a break of three to five hours. Work continued at four or five p.m. and ended between eight and ten p.m. Twelve to 14 hours of work were the rule in Berlin (Möller and Hesselbarth, 1998, p. 104). One nurse of the Diakonia Association who had worked at the Martin Luther Hospital reported in retrospect:

> A 60-hour work week was the standard schedule in patient care, and exceeding this time was something that was not even mentioned. The nurses lived at the hospital; at the Martin Luther Hospital not above the wards, as was common elsewhere, but all together in one of the side wings. That way, they were within reach at any time. Split shifts were taken for granted, and so the nurse was around her patients in the morning and afternoon and, if possible, looked after them every single day.
>
> (Klütz, 1981, pp. 39–48)

All sisterhoods published periodicals in which they provided information about their work. These publications, usually monthly or annual journals, primarily addressed their supporters, because the communities had rather professionally organised departments to collect donations. The nurses' work is discussed in these magazines, but the topic of working conditions is spared. Working hours are only mentioned occasionally: never as a stand-alone subject, but only in connection with a story on caring for a particular patient. In these stories, the workload is always portrayed as something done out of religious motivation; it never appears to be a burden, but rather is seen as a labour of love.

In a publication from 1956, the matron of the sisterhood at the Martin Luther Hospital recalled caring for the homeless at the hospital around 1931, of which the so-called welfare sister (*Fürsorgeschwester*) was in charge:

> Sister Gabriele, our welfare sister, takes care of about 80 to 90 hungry people a day, be it with a bowl of soup or some bread crusts collected on the ward after every meal. In any wind and weather, the starving in their ragged clothes line up in long queues in front of our hospital and wait for the moment when they are given something to eat.
>
> (Lingner, 1956, p. 21)

Were hospitals religious spaces at that time? It is true that 'sisters constructed both medical and sacred space within the environment of the hospital' (Mann Wall, 2011, p. 62). However, this was only the case in the nursing sphere. Hospitals have always been economic spaces, too. Management not only had to negotiate about money with local governments, foundations, consistories and parishes. The communities were also always involved in administration and often did the accounting. Still, it was not part of the nurses' self-concept to speak about financial affairs publicly.

Withdrawal

This system continued until the end of the Second World War. Then something happened which the nursing historian Susanne Kreutzer (2005, p. 8) aptly describes with the following words: 'The demand for nursing care, which was ever-increasing as German society was growing more affluent, could be satisfied less and less, because the traditional model of a "labour of love" was drastically losing its appeal among younger women.'

Fewer and fewer girls and young women were interested in this career. All three former motives were losing their significance: the religious community as a safety net, nursing as one of the few professional careers for women and the religious sense of mission. At the same time, the demand for nurses was rising, because the health sector was constantly growing. The number of hospital beds in the Federal Republic of Germany grew from 545,745 in 1949 to 712,055 in 1979 (Rausch, 1984, p. 111). The hospitals were already dramatically short of nurses by 1950 (Seidler and Leven, 2003, p. 264; Kreutzer, 2005, p. 24). The communities reacted to the shortage in different ways. The hospitals first tried to replace the nurses from the mother-houses with independent secular employees, whether they were qualified nurses or unskilled workers. The four hospitals analysed here also tried this rather forcefully. The most drastic action was taken by the matron of the *Waldkrankenhaus Spandau*. When she heard that new blocks of flats had been built in the vicinity, she posted job offers to each one of the hundreds of new apartments (Tangerding, 2012, p. 104).

Another effort was to build flats for the employees on the hospital grounds or in the nearby area (Kreutzer, 2005, p. 176). Some motherhouses and sisterhoods even tried to reduce the nurses' workload.

In 1954, the superior of the Protestant Diakonia Association was in negotiations with hospital management at the *Waldkrankenhaus Spandau* about payment and working hours for nurses, but management refused to meet any of the demands (Fritz Mieth: Note dated 21.12.1954, Archiv des Evangelischen Diakonievereins Berlin–Zehlendorf, H 630). The way the people in charge handled these negotiations suggests that they were still convinced the shortage of nurses would soon pass. Another example of this hopeful outlook is a statement by the chairman of the hospital's board of trustees Gerhard Jacobi. Jacobi had played an important role within the Confessing Church (*Bekennende Kirche*) between 1933 and 1945 (Wörmann, 1991, p. 141). He compared the self-sacrificing deaconess to the secular nurse who was merely doing her work in an anniversary publication in 1962:

> Faith in the Lord who has sacrificed himself for us should inspire the deaconess to sacrifice herself as well. Her sacrifice is manifold. She does not demand standard wages, she wears her uniform continually (on her holiday, too), which involuntarily imposes on her much renunciation, and not just with regard to fashion, and above all she sacrifices herself for her

sick patients. [. . .] When I was a patient at the Elisabeth Hospital once, I did not succeed, even as chairman of the board, to send the ward sister away at 7:30 p.m. She was still moving from one bed to the next at 8:30 p.m., quite often until 9 p.m., even though she had got up at 5:45 a.m. The deaconess is overexerting herself!

(Jacobi, 1962, p. 15)

Despite all efforts, the number of secular nurses could not meet the growing demand (Kreutzer, 2014, p. 228). Accordingly, many hospitals cast their net wider in the early 1970s and turned to other countries for help. After some difficulties, nurses from South Korea were hired and came to West Germany in large numbers as independent nurses (Schmuhl, 2002, p. 160; Mattes, 2005, p. 201). Their initially only temporary employment was extended indefinitely a few years later, because it soon became obvious that the religious communities were continuing to experience a shortage of young women.

All recruiting efforts by the religious communities proved to be in vain. They had to pull out of hospital care, especially since they were confronted with the new task of caring for the large numbers of their own ageing sisters. The majority of communities terminated their contracts with the hospital operators between the late-1970s and mid-1980s. It was the end of an era which had lasted about 150 years. Hospitals were no longer places of faith, even though they generally kept their devout names. The Diakonia Association withdrew from the Martin Luther Hospital in 1986. At that time, there were still 27 members of the sisterhood working at the hospital, while the total number of employees was 760 (Tangerding, 2011b, p. 74). They had been responsible both for nursing and management from 1931 onwards. The sister-hood of the Protestant Union, who had moved their motherhouse to the Hubertus Hospital after the end of the Second World War, ceased cooperation in 1972 and closed down the nursing school it had operated (Tangerding, 2011a, p. 61). At the Elisabeth Hospital, the retreat happened step by step. The position of superior was abolished in 1962. Until then, he had been part of hospital management. At the same time, the matron as head of nursing was removed and replaced with a secular director of nursing (*Pflegedirektion*; Tangerding, 2012, p. 146). Seven years later, the hospital's corporate body was converted into a foundation with the already existing board of trustees at its head. The former chairman became the chairman of the board of the Association for the Foundation of Protestant Hospitals, which already owned the Martin Luther Hospital and the Hubertus Hospital (Tangerding, 2012, p. 155). Those deaconesses who were still able to work were now taking care of the old and feeble sisters within their own commu-nity. The motherhouse comprised 64 deaconesses in 1968 and 52 of them were older than 65 years (Tangerding, 2012, p. 146). The Diakonia Association only withdrew from the *Waldkrankenhaus Spandau* in 2003. There was no shift from matron to secular director of nursing staff (*Pflegedienstleitung*) like at the other Protestant hospitals, but the last matron additionally adopted the title of director of nursing when she was elected in 1988.

Parallel to the sisterhoods' withdrawal, groups inside the hospitals started to affiliate with the large trade union 'Public Services, Transport and Traffic' (*ÖTV*) and fought for wage settlements. Employee representatives professionalised their work and claimed co-determination in the decision process. Trade unions appeared on the scene at many public hospitals and played an increasing role in decision-making processes. The situation was different in Protestant hospitals.

Superiors of sisterhoods and motherhouses had always negotiated directly with hospital management and the community as a whole. For independent nurses, who over the years had replaced more and more of the affiliated ones, there were no general wage agreements either. Management offered contracts corresponding to wage settlements at the public hospitals. However, hospital leaders did not join the agreements (Gehring and Thiele, 2002, p. 1002). Independent nurses had to accept the contracts offered if they wanted to work at one of these Protestant hospitals. During the withdrawal of the religious communities, the free nurses increasingly acted as replacement staff for the former nurses, and within a short while they were solely responsible for patient care.

Emergence of political engagement

There was only a little political activity at the four Protestant hospitals up to 1972. However, it would be wrong to assert that motherhouses and sisterhoods prevented co-determination. Employees, whether they were affiliated or non-affiliated nurses, did not even demand to be more involved. The retreat of the motherhouses and sisterhoods did not arouse the interest of the secular nurses into fighting with management for their rights. In fact, it was a law in 1972 and the Federal Republic's economic crisis which fanned the flames.

In that year, the German parliament adopted the most influential law on the financing of hospitals after the Second World War: the Law on Hospital Funding (*Krankenhausfinanzierungsgesetz*). To put it simply, with this law, the federal states committed themselves to financing extraordinary investments, such as new facilities, substantial renovations and expensive equipment. However, they would only support those hospitals which had been added to the so-called 'Hospital Plan'. This plan was based on calculations of requirements and general political principles, for example, a diversity of hospital owners (*Trägervielfalt*). The plan was supposed to include public, private and church-run hospitals. Institutions could barely continue to exist without a place on the list. This law, however, did not end the debates on hospital funding. When the rate of unemployment rose and the first oil crisis happened in the early 1970s (Simon, 2000, p. 89), arguments became even more impassioned.

Partly as a reaction to these developments, trade unions and employee representatives at the Protestant hospitals fought for shorter working hours, better pay and collective wage agreements. They demanded that more staff be hired and that they would be involved in the internal decision-making process. Employees often felt that management was willing to make too many trade-offs in order to ensure a position on the new Hospital Plan. Management, on the other hand, often regarded the views of trade unions and employee representatives as far too naive.

The *Waldkrankenhaus Spandau* put a new ward building into operation in 1979. The governing Mayor of Berlin and hundreds of other guests attended the opening ceremony. During the event, a group of employees handed out leaflets to those present. The pamphlet's heading said, 'Behind the new façade':

> Ever-growing numbers of referrals have not been accompanied by creating more positions for nursing staff. As a consequence, there is still no five-day week in the care sector, the wards are on the verge of collapse in winter and when rates of sick leave are high. Operations can only be kept running by working overtime (which in this hospital is not paid properly at all) and by sacrificing spare time on the weekend. [. . .] We have felt compelled to publish this because we believe that pretty speeches during election season are not suitable whatsoever for addressing the specific problems faced by patients and staff.
>
> (Scholz, Kentenich, Brenner, Müller [Mitarbeitervertretung]:
> Wie es hinter der Fassade aussieht. 02.03.1979, Archiv der Paul
> Gerhardt Diakonie, Alte Akte WKH, 7.78–11.79)

For the first time, doctors and nurses at the *Waldkrankenhaus Spandau* were collectively voicing their protest and becoming actively involved as employee representatives side by side. This would not have been possible during the long period of sisterhoods and motherhouses. A similar involvement can also be observed in the case of Peter Reeg at the *Elisabeth Krankenhaus* (Tangerding, 2012, p. 158).

In June 1977, doctor Peter Reeg handed out invitations to a meeting of the trade union *ÖTV*, to which he belonged. The internist, who was also a member of the employee representation at the Elisabeth Hospital, had distributed *ÖTV* papers before. A new intensive care unit had been opened in 1976. The main interest of Reeg and his fellow campaigners was the recruitment of more nurses for intensive care, whereas he viewed the number of doctors as sufficient.

Soon after his latest advertising efforts for the trade union, he received a written note from administrative director Jens-Martin Rudloff: 'The invitation letters you distributed represent an intolerable agitation and call for a labour dispute at the hospital. They grossly violate the preservation of labour peace at our hospital, which cannot be tolerated under any circumstances' (Dokumentation 'Weg mit der Kündigung von Peter Reeg!' 1977, ArchPGD,

Schriftverkehr Vorstand 01.01.1976 – 31.12.1987). The doctor was dismissed without further notice. Reeg took legal action against the dismissal and won the first trial. However, a higher court confirmed the hospital management's standpoint.

At the time, hospital directors were not used to nurses and assistant doctors fighting so vehemently for their rights. How overwhelmed the clinic managers were can be seen from a variety of sources. In 1974, a board member of the Association for the Foundation of Protestant Hospitals in Berlin took the establishment of a local ÖTV labour committee as an opportunity to ask 'whether a clause prohibiting any political and subversive activities in our hospitals should not be included in the employment contracts' (Protokoll der Vorstandssitzung vom 04.12.1974, ArchPGD, Verein Protokolle 1971–1978).

The board member asking the question was Rolf E. Dohrmann, head of the Department of Internal Medicine. At that time, the very same physician agreed to the medical treatment of Irene Goergens, who was an imprisoned member of the Red Army Fraction (*Rote Armee Fraktion*; Tangerding, 2012, p. 122).

The report continues: 'Although all board members agree with the idea, such a step is unanimously viewed as not being legally feasible at this time.'

Clinic managers were now forced to put issues up for discussion. The times when they had decided on matters all by themselves were over. Their decisions could even be reversed. In 1978, the director of the Protestant Hospital Hubertus invited his staff to the annual Christmas party (Tangerding, 2011a, p. 68). Employee representatives refused the invitation and conducted a survey among the staff. They could choose between the following: Christmas party in the old manner, a summer party, no event at all or making their own suggestion. The poll was won by those opposing the traditional Christmas party. A summer party was planned. The medical director, however, objected and pointed out that the grounds were not suitable for outdoor celebrations and patients would be disturbed. The argument wore on. Christmas celebrations were indeed cancelled, but an official summer party did not take place either. In 1979, the clinic no longer extended invitations to a Christmas party, but to a 'pre-Christmas service followed by a casual get-together'. The medical director feared for the hospital's religious image and wrote to the managing director: 'We will surely live to see Christmas parties being held in urban hospitals while we stand on the sidelines' (Tangerding, 2011a, p. 68).

Apart from the fact that employees were fighting for better working conditions in general and demanding democratic procedures, there was a third point of contention, which was the most severe of all: employees were claiming political space. They used the hospital for their demands. Not only staff at the *Waldkrankenhaus Spandau* itself, but also student assistants on night watch at the Hubertus Hospital as well as a few other groups gave out political leaflets to guests, relatives, co-workers and pedestrians. They put up invitations on the noticeboard and organised meetings inside the hospitals. The superior of the Diakonia Association met with representatives of the ÖTV in 1978 to negotiate about political campaigns by the trade union at the Martin Luther

Hospital. As a result, the *ÖTV* was given the right to use the noticeboard in order to keep *ÖTV* members up to date. However, all announcements had to be phrased in a neutral way so as to respect the autonomy of the Church regarding labour law (Hartmut Warns an Wolf Kander am 19.06.1978, Archiv des Martin Luther Krankenhauses Berlin, C 16).

The Protestant hospitals continued to refuse any negotiation of wage agreements with the trade unions and established the so-called 'Third Way'. The Third Way is a concept of the church agencies and assumes that there are no employers and employees in their institutions, but service providers and service takers. It established a board for negotiations between the two parties in which the trade unions did not have a seat. Moreover, it stipulated that it was illegal for service takers to go on strike and for service providers to lock out service takers. Works councils (*Betriebsräte*) were replaced by staff representations (*Mitarbeiterversammlungen*), which were not as influential as the works councils. The Third Way was adopted by the members of the Protestant Church in Germany (*Evangelische Kirche in Deutschland*) in 1979. To a certain extent, and with permission from the management, trade unions, such as the *ÖTV*, remained a presence inside the hospitals. However, due to the restructuring – the Third Way – their activities were severely restricted.

Members of employee representations were elected by the whole staff. However, the few remaining sisters had to abstain from voting, not because staff representatives prohibited it, but because the motherhouses and superiors did not allow them to get involved.

Even as late as 1980, the board of the Protestant Diakonia Association stated:

> that in accordance with the sisterhood's regulations we maintain that our deaconess sisters and students will not participate in the upcoming election of the new employee representative committee, but that they are prepared to play a part in employee representation after the election by sending delegates to work on tasks of mutual interest regarding work at the Martin Luther Hospital.
>
> (Hartmut Warns an Hansjörg Meier-Duis am 12.12.1980, ArchPGD, MLK 80)

Summary

It needs to be noted that there was a huge divide between the religious communities and the politically active staff. The latter did not make any reference to the sisterhoods and motherhouses. They did not break away from them, but rather fought their battles without referring to history or traditions. Their way of living was already so different that it was hardly necessary for them to dissociate themselves.

The separation which had for a long time existed between doctors and nurses was eventually overcome by the members of these two groups. This was certainly restricted to concrete and political activities and did not find its way into the everyday life on the ward. Their common and collective aims served as the main drive towards cooperation.

It is remarkable that the employees made hardly any reference to the patients in their protests. The patients' well-being was pushed to the background. Better working conditions became a value per se. This was a radical departure from the religious communities' principle of serving patients. Declaring political aims at all without considering the patients would not have been possible in any of the four hospitals before the sisterhoods had retreated. Printing political demands onto leaflets and distributing them to fellow employees and passers-by would have been even harder to imagine for a deaconess.

The protests did not erupt because the religious communities had disappeared. However, they were only possible because the deaconesses and members of the Diakonia Association had left. Only with their withdrawal could the space of the hospital become a political one. This happened not only because employees fought for better working conditions, but also because they demanded it publicly. Conflicts with management did not take place behind closed doors. Employee representatives were keen to find suitable ways to publish their demands. Sometimes it was with a leaflet or through an announcement on the noticeboard, other times it was by means of a meeting in a hospital room. In one way or another, the focus of communication had shifted from patients to employees.

The emergence of politics led to a change in self-concept of those who were politically involved. It became part of their profession and their understanding of professionalism to deal with hospital politics, to know the legal differences between Third Way agreements and the unions' wage settlements. They were increasingly knowledgeable about different systems of working hours and fought for their preferred one on the basis of both political convictions and hard facts.

An interesting question to ask is whether professionalism has, to a certain extent, replaced the model of self-sacrifice which had been predominant for nearly 150 years. Understanding nursing as a labour of love rules out any distinct boundaries in terms of space, time, work content and economics. Members of religious communities did, in fact, live side by side with their patients, spent almost all their time caring for them, were engaged in every kind of task which needed to be taken care of and were not directly paid for their efforts. Nursing as a profession, however, comes with clear distinctions relating to all four aspects mentioned. Nurses spend only their working time on the wards, there is a clear separation between working hours and spare time, they are not responsible for every single task on the ward, even though fulfilling a huge and complex range of assignments, and finally, they receive direct payment for their work.

Interestingly, Sr Liliane Juchli, one of the leading figures in nursing care and founder of the nursing model 'Activities of Daily Living', declares professionalism to be one of the two crucial categories for nursing in the twenty-first century. Juchli (1991) argues that after an emphasis on the 'art of nursing'

(*Pflegekunst*) in the Middle Ages and on the 'technique of nursing' (*Pflegetechnik*) from the early modern period until the end of the twentieth century, a new era has begun which she calls the 'study of nursing' (*Pflegekunde*). Founded on a holistic approach to care, it breaks away from a purely science-based concept of nursing. Nevertheless, the era of nursing studies can only be a success if nursing is taught as a profession, not as a service. One can read the following as a call, but also as a comment on the history of nursing (Juchli, 1991, p. 19): 'The mission of nursing care in the 21st century is thereby spelt out: holistic and professional health care and nursing.'

References

Bildstein, K., Groß, D. and Kühl, R., 2009. Betreff meines aerztlichen Gutachtens gebe ich die eidesstattliche Versicherung ab, dasselbe nach bestem Wissen erstattet zu haben. Eugenisch-psychiatrische Anträge an Erbgesundheitsgerichte am Beispiel des Alexianer Krankenhauses Aachen (1934–1939). In: S. Westermann, R. Kühl, D. Groß, eds. *Medizin im Geist der "Erbgesundheit". Beiträge zur Geschichte der Eugenik und "Rassenhygiene"*. Münster: Lit. pp. 39–56.

Bolk, R., 1984. *Das Krankenhaus am Urban. Medizingeschichtliche Untersuchung eines Krankenhauses der Stadt Berlin 1887–1945*. Berlin/Bonn: Westkreuz.

Bowen, G.A., 2009. Document Analysis as a Qualitative Research Method. *Qualitative Research Journal*, 9(2), pp. 27–40.

Breiding, B., 1998. *Die Braunen Schwestern: Ideologie, Struktur, Funktion einer national-sozialistischen Elite*. Stuttgart: F. Steiner.

Gehring, H. and Thiele, C., 2002. Kirchenarbeitsrecht. In: H. Schliemann, ed. *Das Arbeitsrecht im BGB*. Berlin: De Gruyter, pp. 978–1122.

Gossner, J., 1849. Untitled. In: Curatorium des Frauen-Kranken-Vereins und Elisabeth-Krankenhauses, ed. *16. Jahresbericht des Frauen-Kranken-Vereins 1848*. Berlin: s.n. [self-published], p. 3.

Jacobi, G., 1962. Die Mutterhaus-Diakonie 1837 und 1962. In: W. Augustat, ed. *125 Jahre Elisabeth-Diakonissen- und Krankenhaus in Berlin*. Berlin: s.n., pp. 13–39.

Juchli, S., 1991. *Krankenpflege. Praxis und Theorie der Gesundheitsförderung und Pflege Kranker*. New York: Thieme, p. 19.

Käppeli, S., 2004. *Vom Glaubenswerk zur Pflegewissenschaft: Geschichte des Mit-Leidens in der christlichen, jüdischen und freiberuflichen Krankenpflege*. Bern: Huber.

Kaufmann, F.-X., 2003. *Der deutsche Sozialstaat im internationalen Vergleich*. Frankfurt/Main: Suhrkamp.

Keller, R., 2007. *Diskursforschung. Eine Einführung für SozialwissenschaftlerInnen*. Wiesbaden: Verlag für Sozialwissenschaften.

Klütz, A., 1981. 50 Jahre Krankenpflege. In: Martin Luther Krankenhaus ed. *50 Jahre Martin-Luther-Krankenhaus*. Berlin: s.n. [self-published], pp. 39–48.

Kreutzer, S., 2005. *Vom "Liebesdienst" zum modernen Frauenberuf. Die Reform der Krankenpflege nach 1945*. Frankfurt/Main: Campus.

Kreutzer, S., 2008. 'Before, we were always there – now, everything is separate': On nursing reforms in Western Germany. *Nursing History Review*, 16, pp. 180–200.

Kreutzer, S., 2014. *Arbeits- und Lebensalltag evangelischer Krankenpflege. Organisation, soziale Praxis und biographische Erfahrungen 1945–1980*. Göttingen: V & R.

Landwehr, A., 2008. *Historische Diskursanalyse*. Frankfurt/Main: Campus.

Lingner, L., 1956. Aus der Chronik des Martin-Luther-Krankenhauses. In: F. Mieth, W. Schian, eds. *Krankendienst im Zeichen des Kreuzes.* Berlin: s.n. [self-published], pp. 21–140.

Mann Wall, B., 2011. Body, Soul, and Service. Catholic–Sister Nurses in Late Nineteenth and Early Twentieth Century Hospitals. In: Patricia D'Antonio, Sandra B. Lewensen, eds. *History as Evidence. Nursing Interventions Through Time,* New York: Springer, pp. 61–74.

Mattes, M., 2005. *"Gastarbeiterinnen" in der Bundesrepublik: Anwerbepolitik, Migration und Geschlecht in den 50er bis 70er Jahren.* Frankfurt/Main: Campus.

Mayring, P., 2000. Qualitative content analysis. *Forum Qualitative Sozialforschung / Forum Qualitative Social Research*, 1. Avaliable through: <www.qualitative-research. net/index.php/fqs/article/view/1089/2386> [accessed 11 August 2015].

McLeod, H., 1982. Protestantism and the working class in imperial Germany. *European Studies Review*, 12, pp. 323–44.

Möller, U. and Hesselbarth, U., 1998. *Die geschichtliche Entwicklung der Krankenpflege. Hintergründe – Analysen – Perspektiven.* Hagen: Kunz.

Nipperdey, T., 1988. *Religion im Umbruch: Deutschland 1870–1918.* Münich: C.H. Beck.

Rapley, T., 2007. *Doing Conversation, Discourse and Document Analysis.* London: Sage.

Rausch, R., 1984. *Die freigemeinnützigen Krankenhäuser in der Bundesrepublik Deutschland. Entwicklungen, Lage, Leistungen und Zukunftsaussichten.* Stuttgart: Bleicher.

Schmuhl, H.-W., 2002. *Evangelische Krankenhäuser und die Herausforderung der Moderne.* Wolfgang Helbig, ed. Leipzig: *Evangelische Verlagsanstalt.*

Schwarz, J., 1998. *Beruf: Schwester. Mutterhausdiakonie im 19. Jahrhundert.* Frankfurt/ Main: Campus.

Schweikardt, C., 2004. Entwicklungen und Trends in der deutschen Krankenpflege-Geschichtsschreibung des 19. und 20. Jahrhunderts. *Medizinhistorisches Journal*, 39(2/3), pp. 197–218.

Seidler, E. and Leven, K.-H., 2003. *Geschichte der Medizin und der Krankenpflege.* Stuttgart: Kohlhammer.

Simon, M., 2000. *Krankenhauspolitik in der Bundesrepublik Deutschland: historische Entwicklung und Probleme der politischen Steuerung stationärer Krankenversorgung.* Opladen: Springer.

Tangerding, C., 2011a. *Geschichte des Evangelischen Krankenhauses Hubertus Berlin.* Paul Gerhardt Diakonie, ed. Berlin: s.n. [self-published].

Tangerding, C., 2011b. *Geschichte des Martin Luther Krankenhauses Berlin.* Paul Gerhardt Diakonie, ed. Berlin: s.n. [self-published].

Tangerding, C., 2012. *Geschichte der Evangelischen Elisabeth Klinik.* Paul Gerhardt Diakonie, ed. Berlin: s.n. [self-published].

Tangerding, C., 2015. Evangelische Krankenfürsorge? Zur Rolle der Konfession im Berliner Krankenhausbau der Weimarer Republik. *Medizin, Gesellschaft und Geschichte*, 33, pp. 65–90.

Virchow, R. (1869). Die berufsmäßige Ausbildung zur Krankenpflege auch außerhalb der bestehenden kirchlichen Organisationen. In: Die Berliner Frauen-Vereins-Conferenz from 5–6 November 1869, pp. 84–93. In: B. Panke-Kochinke, ed. 2000. *Die Geschichte der Krankenpflege (1679–2000). Ein Quellenbuch.* Frankfurt/Main: Mabuse, pp. 64–8.

von Rotenhan, W., 1962. Die Geschichte des Hauses. Bericht zur Hundertjahrfeier 1937. In: W. Augustat, ed. *125 Jahre Elisabeth-Diakonissen- und Krankenhaus in Berlin.* Berlin: s.n. [self-published], pp. 52–76.

Wolff, H.-P. and Wolff, J., 1994. *Geschichte der Krankenpflege*. Basel: Recom.

Wolff, H.-P. and Wolff, J., 2002. *Studien zur deutschsprachigen Geschichte der Pflege*. Frankfurt/Main: Mabuse.

Wörmann, H.-W., 1991. *Widerstand in Charlottenburg. Heft 5 der Schriftenreihe über den Widerstand in Berlin 1933–1945*. Gedenkstätte Deutscher Widerstand, ed. Berlin: s.n. [self-published].

Zerull, L.M., 2011. Filling the Gaps in Community Care: Parish Nurses Working Out of Congregations. In: P. D'Antonio and S.B. Lewensen, eds. *History as Evidence. Nursing Interventions Through Time*. New York: Springer, ch. 7.

3 How to write a letter

A physician's letters from the viewpoint of medical humanities

Katharina Fürholzer

Medical authorship

What is a physician? I would say one part of being a physician is being a writer. After all, working in a hospital environment makes authorship an integral part of the medical profession. One may just think of scientific articles, reviews, expert opinions, medical reports or case studies as ways to step into a written exchange with colleagues, insurance companies or legislative authorities. Communicating on a written basis, therefore, forms an essential part of a physician's day-to-day obligations, both in research and in clinical practice. Fortunately, profound communication skills, especially when it comes to doctor–patient relationships, are considered a key feature of modern medical professionalism, which has already had sustainable effects on the academic education of medical students. Nowadays, more and more universities not only teach the multifaceted challenge of doctor–patient interactions within lecture rooms, but also provide their students with the opportunity to practise professional communication competences within specially designed skills labs, allowing them, for example, to 'break bad news' under protected conditions and with differentiated feedback before being confronted with the authentic setting of the hospital. Whereas *spoken* communication is firmly anchored in the curriculum of medical students, the relevance, ability and skill of *written* communication as an equally constitutive part of the medical profession is still widely neglected in theory and practice. The following chapter elaborates on this subject with examples of probably the most important means of written communication within the doctor–patient relationship: the genre of a physician's letters, commonly better known as discharge summaries.[1] The aim of the chapter is to approach some of the conflicts that can arise when physicians communicate via letter both with other physicians and with patients, in order to finally highlight the – also ethically significant – effects of the *author–reader* relationship on the *doctor–patient* relationship.

Writing a physician's letters: theory and practice

Content and structure

Letters result from a doctor's professional task of observing, assessing and interpreting symptoms and patients' reports, of depicting information that is of particular relevance and of arranging and weighing the data collected in order to elucidate what is important and why.[2] The effective structure, content and scope of letters are not standardised (Book, 2011, p. 20), however, including information on the following has been recommended for the last few decades:

- *medical encounters*: principal, secondary, differential diagnoses;
- *medical history*: reason for admission or referral, diagnosis applicable at the time of admission; medication and medical allergies; family and social history;
- *examinations and investigations*: vital signs (blood pressure, heart rate); physical and psychological examination findings; laboratory and X-ray reports;
- *medications and therapy*: operational, psychotherapeutic and pharmacological treatment (drug name and dosage); possible check-ups;
- *impression*: case summary; prognosis; ability to work; patient's level of information or understanding.[3]

Functions and criticism

The specific function assigned to a letter depends on its respective addressee (Glazinski, 2007, pp. 26–40). It might be helpful for matters of differentiation to heuristically cluster a letter's possible receivers into the trinomial reader-model of the explicit reader, implied reader and the actual or real reader:[4]

- *explicit reader(s)*: people or institutions addressed directly by the writer;
- *implied reader(s)*: other people or institutions the writer had in mind while writing but which are not addressed explicitly within the text;
- *actual or real reader(s)*: all people who actually read the text whether the writer had them in mind or not.

With regard to a letter's implied readers, the requirements are as huge and versatile as the group itself, as a letter can be directed implicitly to cost units, courts, public prosecutors, social agencies, annuity insurances, health insurances, statisticians, the patient's employers or authorised experts, to name just a few (Hausner, Hajak and Spießl, 2008, p. A 27). The main function of a physician's letters, however, is linked with their explicit readers, namely the referring physician, the general practitioner and the specialist; within these internal doctor–doctor relationships, letters mainly serve the classical and legally mandatory purpose of transmitting medically relevant data for subsequent patient care and, thus, to inform about examinations carried out, diagnoses that were made, subsequent treatment steps or prescribed medications (Walraven and Rokosh, 1999, p. 160; Glazinski, 2007, pp. 25–8; Hausner *et al.*, 2008, p. A 27; Jauch, 2013, pp. 787–8). Furthermore, as many registered doctors consider letters as an important means of training, they are also supposed to provide information on new diagnostic and therapeutic developments (for example, Heckl, 1990, p. 7). It is the physician's task to have all those different readers and correlating claims in view, in order to provide each addressee with exactly the kinds of information needed.

With regard to points of criticism within written doctor–doctor communication, the average time of transmission, the level of content and the general quality of letters are considered particularly problematic. In the opinion of most physicians, having to wait more than a fortnight renders letters useless, as at this point in time, further treatment has usually already started (Spießl and Cording, 2001, p. 186). Nevertheless, the majority of referring physicians complain about receiving letters only after an average of two to four weeks, and some have to wait even up to six months (Spießl and Cording, 2001, p. 185). Preliminary discharge letters with basic information on diagnoses, findings and therapeutic measures are supposed to reduce the conflicts that accompany delays in letter transmissions (Book, 2011, pp. 20–1). Whether they are actually read in the end, however, is another question: According to a German study carried out in 2001, only 17 per cent of general practitioners read over 75 per cent of a letter's content (Spießl and Cording, 2001, p. 184).[5] This low rate might come as less of a surprise when the fact that general practitioners receive an average of ten letters a day is taken into account (Spießl and Cording, 2001, p. 184).

Regarding content, the amount of information provided is usually perceived as too low or vague. This starts with popular phrases such as 'we kindly presume you are familiar with the patient's history', which can be seen as a disregard of the significance and complexity of medical case histories; one must not forget the huge amount of patient information any physician is supposed to correctly and immediately have on call (Heckl, 1990, p. 16; Glazinski, 2007, p. 39). Additionally, many practitioners find explanations of diagnosis and prognosis inaccurate (Heckl, 1990, pp. 6, 88–9). Information and recommendations regarding current or prospective therapy and medication are commonly estimated as limited, circumstantial or impractical; the patients' knowledge of their condition is often not mentioned at all (Heckl, 1990, p. 87; Spießl and Cording, 2001, p. 185).

Eventually, the common linguistic and stylistic uncleanliness of letters is also a constant bone of contention. To this day, little has changed in doctors' characteristic predilection for passive constructions, nominal style, hypotactic sentences and abundant changes of tense (Neumann-Mangoldt, 1964, pp. 23–6; Glazinski, 2007, p. 36). Moreover, the extensive accumulation of technical terms and abbreviations usually only familiar in one single speciality makes letters even harder to understand – even for medical specialists. Considering that letters often constitute the sole contact between hospitalists and practitioners and that comprehension difficulties might have an immediate effect on the patient in the form of unnecessary tests, delayed diagnosis, intermittent treatment and increased complications (Spießl and Cording, 2001,

p. 184; Book, 2011, p. 21; see also Epstein, 1995), adequate medical mail communication is crucial.[6]

Teaching physician's letters: learning by doing

Despite the important and complex meaning of a physician's letters, the correct placement of their structure, content and function in correlation with explicit and implied addressees is a more than marginal issue within regular medical training. Considering that even in 2001, approximately 45,000 letters left German hospitals every day, meaning that every hospital doctor had to invest an average of three hours a day in this legally binding task (Spießl, 2001, p. A 2568; Glazinski, 2007, p. 30), it seems even more fatal that how to write a letter is still not systematically taught (Jauch, 2013, p. 787). This deficit has been rendered problematic by the medical world for quite some time: in the early 1960s, Peter Neumann-Mangoldt described the insecurities a young intern or resident can be faced with: 'What kind of results should he disclose and which was he allowed to leave out? Was it appropriate to write within a certain order? Were there any binding rules under which a physician's letter should be written down?' (Neumann-Mangoldt, 1964, p. 2 [Translation KF]). The lack of (theoretical) processing and (practical) teaching of a physician's letters is not limited to the German national borders; to get an inkling of the scale of the issue, one can just look as an example at a 2012 account of the situation in Australia: 'the process of communication at the interface between general practice and hospital has remained unchanged for decades. Yet letter writing is not formally taught in undergraduate or postgraduate medical courses' (Jiwa and Dhaliwal, 2012, p. 40). Under these circumstances, it is not really surprising that the complaints mentioned about communication problems are inevitable. Roughly speaking, 'learning by doing' is the simple way that the issue of teaching letter writing is normally tackled (Erdogan-Griese, 2010, p. 23). Due to the absence of structured assistance or guidance, many young doctors orient themselves to copies of former letters or discuss first writing attempts with experienced colleagues (Krusche, 1976, p. 216; Müller, Löll and Bechtold, 2008, p. 25); in addition, a negligible number of medical books offer guidance that is oftentimes limited to only a few pages or even lines (Book, 2011, p. 20). However, this does not really solve the overall problem, as Book puts it in a nutshell: 'Generally applicable standards are [. . .] neither to be found in the curriculum of medical studies nor in medical textbooks' (Book, 2011, p. 20 [Translation KF]).

Writer–reader relationships: patients as readers

How letters are commonly taught and written turns into an ethical issue when taking another reader into account not mentioned so far: the patients themselves. Patients are oftentimes not necessarily seen as problematic – after all, they are not the addressee or what we call the explicit or maybe even implied reader. Patients' access to 'their' letters is not uniformly regulated in Germany. In theory, according to legislators, every patient has a right to inspect the files – and, thus, also letters – concerning his or her case (Hausner *et al.*, 2008). In practice, the ways of supplying patients with letter-based information about their diagnosis, treatment and prognosis are up to the respective hospital, ward or the attending physician; practices range from delivering either copies or originals to patients, either in an open or sealed envelope, up to cases in which patients do not get their hands on their letters at all, as those are sent directly to the referring doctor (for example, Spießl, 2001, p. A 2568). Whereas in spoken communication, physicians are normally just confronted with meeting the expectations and needs of one singular person or group, in written letters, the multifaceted needs of all different addressees come together in one single place. In addition, having to deal with the particular needs of vulnerable patients in this conglomerate of demands poses an immense challenge. After all, the letter writer has to juggle with quite opposing information requirements:

* information the patient wants to know;
* information the patient does not want to know;
* information the doctor does not want the patient to know;
* information the doctor wants the patient to know.

It may, thus, not come as much of a surprise that many doctors have solid concerns about whether supplying patients with letters is actually for their own good. While many practitioners agree that providing patients with letters can serve as a useful reminder of the former consultations and decisions, promoting patient understanding and involvement, consequently, leading to increased trust, better communication and improved doctor–patient relationships (Morrow *et al.*, 2005; Baxter *et al.*, 2008, p. 260), there are equally weighted concerns that patients might, in fact, have great difficulties understanding medical terminology and that letters can cause worry or distress, especially where there is bad news or where serious symptoms or multiple possible diagnoses are described in the text (Morrow *et al.*, 2005; Baxter *et al.*, 2008, p. 260).

Regardless of whether one is in favour of supplying patients with letters or not, adhering to the current law and common practice, most patients receive letters and, thus, potentially read them. For medical practices, this means that doctor–patient relationships expand to a written level. As soon as patients read letters, they have both the role of a patient and a reader, and the letter writer is, at the same time, both writer and physician. When communicating by letters, there is, thus, an inseparable simultaneity of the doctor–patient relationship and the writer–reader relationship. For physicians, speaking to their patients also on a written level means that, in addition to the ethical commitment entailed by the medical profession, they also have an ethical responsibility as writers.

(Ethical) implications: medium and genre

In order to raise awareness among medical students and doctors that the expansion of 'classic' medical communication on a written level may have – also ethically relevant – effects on the overall doctor–patient relationship, it might be of use to look at two exemplary aspects of letters: their medium and their genre.

Medium: written vs. spoken language

It sounds quite banal, but, first of all, a letter is a medium of written language. Within our sociocultural context, that which is written is basically associated with a higher degree of distance: while sender and receiver within spoken interactions usually stand within a temporal or spatial proximity, written messages are normally exchanged with a certain intermittence (Koch and Oesterreicher, 1985, p. 19). This distance between sender and receiver and, thus, the conditions of exchange, contribute to a more monologic mode of communicating, whereas orality allows for an immediate change of speaker roles (Koch and Oesterreicher, 1985, pp. 19–23). It is this proximity between sender and receiver that makes spoken language more spontaneous, expressive and affective (Koch and Oesterreicher, 1985, p. 23; Dürscheid, 2006, p. 30).

In reference to written doctor–patient communication, there is one property of literacy that is of particular importance: finality. Scripture outlasts time, and this allows one to trace back its individual historicity. What is put down in written words is estimated as more durable, as less easily revisable than spoken language, which is usually characterised as being bound to presence, as being volatile (Koch and Oesterreicher, 1985, pp. 21–3; Dürscheid, 2006, p. 26). We commonly regard literacy as the language of experts, while, by contrast, spoken language is linked more with the laity (for example, Raible, 1994, p. 1). As such, we associate the language of experts with a significant higher truth – just because of its medium. With regard to the medical context, this poses the risk that, due to its written mediality, a letter is attributed with a higher degree of truth than the preceding oral doctor–patient consultation or even conceived as an incontrovertible truth – notwithstanding that the letter writer did not perhaps intend to state hard and non–negotiable facts at all, but meant rather to record hypotheses, potentialities or situational and subjective suspicions, expressed, for example, by differential diagnoses. That a letter should not be perceived as a 1:1 depiction of reality also becomes obvious when considering to what degree a letter's final structure and content is influenced by the multitude of explicit and implied addressees and corresponding functions.[7] However, before turning to the specific – especially ethical – meaning of the aspects of literacy, we should first question what kind of genre a letter actually corresponds to. Or, to put it into simpler words: what exactly is a letter?

Genre: letters and biographies

At first glance, questioning a letter's genre may seem a bit redundant as well; after all, the 'architextual' assignment of the letter, meaning the taxonomic relation of a text with a genre or genres (Genette, 1992),[8] is already heralded by its name. Further clear markers for the letter genre are its materiality – we have the envelope, the loose pages (instead of, for example, a casebound novel or a printed comic) – as a part of a genre's paratext, thus, everything that surrounds a text's main body.[9] Other paratextual signs are typical formalities, such as address fields, conventional salutations, reference lines, place and date, logos and so on. With regard to the specific conditions of our context, some particular features can be discerned that separate medical letter writing from the conventions of the overall genre. Difficulties arise, for instance, in linking the letter's content with one clear voice: Within the German system, a physician's letters do not usually reveal who is actually speaking: within letters' jargon and form, identity-establishing first person pronouns seem quite frowned upon, suggesting facticity rather than subjectivity (for example, Donnelly, 1997); writer-identifying signature fields also usually contain the names of several people (chief physician, attending physician, resident), effectively assigning authorship not to a single writer but to a medical collective. Beyond that, correspondence within medical letter communication is not usually reciprocal, meaning there is no mutual exchange of messages (Hamann, 2001, p. 149); this enforces the medical collective's monologic style and the medium-associated connotation of truth and finality.

Even though the text, form and function of a letter allow for a certain architextual approach, on closer inspection, the physician's letter's specific mode of being seems to be way more than 'just' a letter. So what exactly is it then? Within the medical system, one might say that a letter is, first and foremost, a conglomerate of two genres: the genre of letter and the genre of biography, or, to be more precise, of the biographical subform of pathography. Anne Hunsaker Hawkins defines pathographies as 'a form of autobiography or biography that describes personal experiences of illness, treatment, and sometimes death' (Hawkins, 1999, p. 1). According to Hawkins, who focuses on autobiographies in her remarks, pathographies symbolise

> the attempts of individuals to orient themselves in the world of sickness [. . .], to achieve a new balance between self and reality, to arrive at an objective relationship both to experience and to the experiencing self. The task of the author of a pathography is not only to describe this disordering process but also to restore to reality its lost coherence and to discover, or create, a meaning that can bind it together again.
>
> (Hawkins, 1999, pp. 2–3)

Regarding the hospital setting, Hawkins considers medical forms of documentation as a sort of counterpart to pathographies: Composed as 'brief factual statements about present symptoms and body chemistry' (Hawkins, 1999, p. 13), the mere purpose of medical reports was to record diagnosis and treatment, whereas Hawkins sees pathographies as extended narratives that focus on the emotional components of a medical experience, situating the illness experience within a person's life and the meaning of that life. When it comes to a physician's letters, I would argue, however, that this specific kind of medical report exceeds pure objective coverage, bearing fundamental features of pathography. As a biographical description focused on a subject reduced to his or her role as a sick person, letters mirror the medical writer's task to interpret symptoms, define illness and restore health, in order to give meaning to a borderline situation of human existence. Letters are, thus, the result of interpreting – interpreting symptoms, patient speech, examination findings and so on – as well as of selecting, arranging and weighing the information and data collected – and from this, what the individual physician estimates as noteworthy. It is this process which makes writing a letter a highly subjective genre. Aiming to capture a patient's experience of a diffuse, vague and confusing existential crisis by giving it a clear name, letters not only serve the purpose of describing so-called facts, but, as Hawkins calls it, restore just like pathographies 'to reality its lost coherence and [. . .] discover, or create, a meaning that can bind it together again'. In doing so, a physician's letters – similar to pathographies – contribute significantly to constituting an (illness) identity – an identity which, according to the implications of literacy in its written version, implies a final truth.

Consequences: identity, autonomy and will

Due to their comparatively lower level of experience and expertise, it can be rather hard for patients to classify properly the letter's consolidated version of their illness and, subsequently, ascribed (illness) identity. One must consider, moreover, that letters might be attributed to a more normative and truer status than (former) spoken consultations because of written language's implication of finality, expertise and truth. There is, thus, a higher probability that patients adopt a potentially hypothetic illness narrative as their own. In a way, letters may stabilise or even constitute how patients 'interpret' their illness identity. In contrast to volatile and present-bound spoken consultations, written texts enable patients to read their own 'story' over and over again and to interpret former, present and future incidents, symptoms or other observations according to the version manifested in the letter. The written text allows internalising of its content, thereby enabling patients to reconstruct a supposedly clear case both in front of their social environment and during subsequent consultations with referring doctors. Additional facets or alternative ways of representing the patient's case may fade into the background – posing the risk that letters turn into self-repeating and perhaps also self-fulfilling prophecies. If the letter's content is not marked as at least the partial result of the medical writer's interpretive skills, in a way this poses a certain conflict with the will and autonomy of the patient; after all, it seems rather questionable to which degree the alleged will is formed by the pathographical act. When patients are not being made aware of the role letters might play in the constitution of an (illness) identity, it has, thus, to be asked whether current practices of written doctor–patient communication really justify speaking of what is actually called an 'informed consent'. Therefore, it is high time to raise awareness of the possible correlations between written and spoken doctor–patient interactions, as equally trained communication skills in both means of expression are vital for today's understanding of medical professionalism. Against this background, it seems a step in the right direction to open the medical and medical ethical discussion regarding the complex art of writing letters.

Notes

1 As I specifically refer to the situation within Germany (even though large parts are probably congruent with other healthcare systems), I chose to use the term 'physician's letters' (instead of 'discharge summaries') as the literal translation of the German word *Arztbriefe*. Additionally, I concentrate on letters written within the hospital setting.

2 As an informative and accurate summary can only be created on the basis of thorough notes, recording patient encounters on a day-to-day basis is almost as important as letter writing itself (many thanks to Christopher Yu for this observation).

3 See, for example, Neumann-Mangoldt, 1964, p. 16; Heckl, 1990, pp. 8–16; Gaus, 2005, pp. 289–90; Glazinski, 2007, pp. 14–15, 43; Müller *et al.*, 2008, p. 25; Jauch, 2013, p. 788.

4 For historic and systematic forms, theories and models of readers and recipients, see, for example, Willand, 2014.

5 Twenty-eight per cent of general practitioners read less than 25 per cent of the letter, 9 per cent read 25–50 per cent and 16 per cent of them read 50–75 per cent (Spießl and Cording, 2001, p. 184).

6 The practices of transmission, reception, content, language or style described are not only rendered problematic in Germany, but are the subject of global criticism (see for example Tulloch *et al.*, 1975; Mageean, 1986; Jacobs and Pringle, 1990; Westerman *et al.*, 1990; Adams, Poskitt and Bristol, 1993; Epstein, 1995; Graham and Wilson, 1997; Linné and Rössner, 2000; DeAngelis, 2010; Jiwa and Dhaliwal, 2012).

7 If we take insurance companies as an example, letters serve, for instance, as a common basis for calculations and reimbursements according to the classification system of diagnosis-related groups (for example, Jauch, 2013, pp. 787–8). Patients are classified within this system under a particular group with similar requirements regarding hospital resources in order to determine the cost of a treatment not case-based, but correspondent to the group assigned. With regards to letters, it is quite a common practice to put profit-yielding diagnosis-related group codes just on the right spot or to give certain weight to principal and secondary diagnoses not only for medical, but also economic reasons.

8 '[T]he entire set of general or transcendental categories – types of discourse, modes of enunciation, literary genres – from which emerges a singular text' (Genette, 1997a, p. 1).

9 '[A] text rarely appears in its naked state, without the reinforcement and accompaniment of a certain number of productions, themselves verbal or not, like an author's name, a title, a preface, illustrations. [...] This accompaniment, of varying size and style, constitutes [...] the paratext of the work' (Genette, 1997b, p. 261).

References

Adams, D.C.R, Poskitt, K.R. and Bristol, J.B., 1993. Surgical discharge summaries. Improving the record. *Annals of the Royal College of Surgeons of England*, 75(2), pp. 96–9.

Baxter, S., Farrell, K., Brown, C., Clarke, J. and Davies, H., 2008. Where have all the copy letters gone? A review of current practice in professional–patient correspondence. *Patient Education and Counseling*, 71(2), pp. 259–64.

Book, K., 2011. *Die Funktion des Entlassungsberichts für die psychosoziale Betreuung von Tumorpatienten an der Schnittstelle zwischen stationärer und ambulanter Versorgung*. Bamberg: Bamberg Universität, Dissertation.

DeAngelis, A.F., 2010. The accuracy of medical history information in referral letters. *Australian Dental Journal*, 55(2), pp. 188–92.

Donnelly, W.J., 1997. Lingua Medica. The language of medical case histories. *Annals of Internal Medicine*, 127(11), pp. 1045–8.

Dürscheid, C., 2006. *Einführung in die Schriftlinguistik*. 3rd ed. Göttingen: Vandenhoeck & Ruprecht.

Epstein, R.M., 1995. Communication between primary care physicians and consultants. *Archives of Family Medicine*, 4(5), pp. 403–9.

Erdogan-Griese, B., 2010. Arztbrief. Mehr als eine ungeliebte Pflicht. *Rheinisches Ärzteblatt*, 12, pp. 23–4.

Gaus, W., 2005. *Dokumentations- und Ordnungslehre. Theorie und Praxis des Information-Retrieval*. 5th ed. Berlin, Heidelberg and New York: Springer.

Genette, G., 1992. *The architext. An introduction*. Translated by J.E. Lewin. Berkeley: University of California Press.

Genette, G., 1997a. *Palimpsests. Literature on the second degree*. Translated by C. Newmann and C. Doubinsky. Lincoln: University of Nebraska Press.

Genette, G., 1997b. Introduction to the paratext. Translated by M. Maclean. *New Literary History*, 22(2), pp. 261–72.

Glazinski, R., 2007. *Arztbriefe optimal gestalten. Leitfaden zur Erstellung qualifizierter ärztlicher Berichte in Klinik und Praxis*. Eschborn: Brainwave Wissenschaftsverlag.

Graham, P.H. and Wilson, G., 1998. Letters from the radiation oncologist. Do referring doctors give a damn? *Australasian Radiology*, 42(3), pp. 222–4.

Hamann, U., 2001. Gynäkologie und Geburtshilfe. In: M. Dorfmüller, ed. 2001. *Die ärztliche Sprechstunde. Arzt, Patient und Angehörige im Gespräch*. Landsberg a. L.: ecomed. pp. 117–49.

Hausner, H., Hajak, G. and Spießl, H., 2008. Krankenunterlagen. Wer darf Einsicht nehmen? *Deutsches Ärzteblatt*, 105(1–2), pp. A 27–9.

Hawkins, A.H., 1999. *Reconstructing illness. Studies in pathography*. 2nd ed. West Lafayette, OH: Purdue University Press.

Heckl, R.W., 1990. *Der Arztbrief. Eine Anleitung zum klinischen Denken*. 2nd ed. Stuttgart and New York: Georg Thieme.

Jacobs, L.G.H. and Pringle, M.A., 1990. Referral letters and replies from orthopaedic departments. Opportunities missed. *British Medical Journal*, 301(6750), pp. 470–3.

Jauch, K.W., 2013. Dokumentation, Arztbrief und Operationsbericht. In: K.W. Jauch, W. Mutschler, J.N. Hoffmann and K.G. Kanz, eds. 2013. *Chirurgie Basisweiterbildung. In 100 Schritten durch den Common Trunk*. 2nd ed. Berlin and Heidelberg: Springer. pp. 787–92.

Jiwa, M. and Dhaliwal, S., 2012. Referral writer: preliminary evidence for the value of comprehensive referral letters. *Quality in Primary Care*, 20(1), pp. 39–45.

Koch, P. and Oesterreicher, W., 1985. Sprache der Nähe – Sprache der Distanz. Mündlichkeit und Schriftlichkeit im Spannungsfeld von Sprachtheorie und Sprachgeschichte. *Romanistisches Jahrbuch*, 36, pp. 15–43.

Krusche, G., 1976. *Der Arztbrief. Probleme zwischenärztlicher Kommunikation am Beispiel des internistischen Arztbriefes.* Munich: Universität, Dissertation.

Linné, Y. and Rössner, S., 2000. Referral letters to an obesity unit. Relationship between doctor and patient information. *International Journal of Obesity*, 24(10), pp. 1379–80.

Mageean, R.J., 1986. Study of 'discharge communications' from hospital. *British Medical Journal (Clinical Research Edition)*, 293(6557), pp. 1281–4.

Morrow, G., Robson, A., Harrington, B. and Haining, S., 2005. A qualitative study to investigate why patients accept or decline a copy of their referral letter from their GP. *British Journal of General Practice*, 55(517), pp. 626–9.

Müller, C., Löll, C. and Bechtold, H., 2008. *Klinikleitfaden für alle Stationen. Leitsymptome – Krankheitsbilder – Praxistipps.* 3rd ed. Munich: Elsevier, Urban & Fischer.

Neumann-Mangoldt, P., 1964. *Der Arztbrief. Eine Fibel zum praktischen Gebrauch.* Munich and Berlin: Urban & Schwarzenberg.

Raible, W., 1994. Allgemeine Aspekte von Schrift und Schriftlichkeit/General aspects of writing and its use. In: H. Günther and O. Ludwig, eds. *Schrift und Schriftlichkeit/ Writing and its use. Ein Interdisziplinäres Handbuch internationaler Forschung/An interdisciplinary handbook of international research.* 1. Halfvol. Berlin and New York: Walter de Gruyter, pp. 1–17.

Spießl, H., 2001. Der Kurzarztbrief. Zeitgewinn. *Deutsches Ärzteblatt*, 99(xx), p. A 2568.

Spießl, H. and Cording, C., 2001. Kurz, strukturiert und rasch übermittelt. Der 'optimale' Arztbrief. *Deutsche Medizinische Wochenschrift*, 126(7), pp. 184–7.

Tulloch, A.J., Fowler, G.H., McMullan, J.J. and Spence, J.M., 1975. Hospital discharge reports. Content and design. *British Medical Journal*, 4(5994), pp. 443–6.

Walraven, C.V. and Rokosh, E., 1999. What is necessary for high-quality discharge summaries? *American Journal of Medical Quality*, 14(4), pp. 160–9.

Westerman, R.F., Hull, F.M., Bezemer, P.D. and Gort, G., 1990. A study of communication between general practitioners and specialists. *British Journal of General Practice*, 40(340), pp. 445–9.

Willand, M., 2014. *Lesermodelle und Lesertheorien. Historische und systematische Perspektiven.* Berlin and Boston: Walter de Gruyter.

Part II

Learning and teaching healthcare professionalism

4 Collaborative decision-making

A normative synthesis of decision-making models in healthcare

Sarah Berger, Cornelia Mahler, Jobst-Hendrik Schultz, Joachim Szecsenyi and Katja Götz

Decision-making and collaborative practice

Although the health professions are prepared educationally for different scopes of practice, teaching decision-making – the process of clinical reasoning and problem-solving – is a common curricular aspect with the focus tailored for each specific discipline according to the legal and regulatory frameworks governing that profession's practice. Clinical reasoning, for example, is taught in nursing (Kuiper, Pesut and Kautz, 2009; Hicks, Geist and House, 2013), physiotherapy (Hendrick *et al.*, 2009), occupational therapy (Neistadt and Atkins, 1996) and also in medicine, where diagnostic reasoning for clinical practice is emphasised (Elstein and Schwarz, 2002; Arocha, Wang and Patel, 2005). Educators support students to think about their own cognitive processes in the steps of clinical decision-making, such as recognising patterns based on knowledge and clinical data, forming hypotheses, critical reflection and problem-solving, and drawing conclusions by applying formal reasoning strategies (Hendrick *et al.*, 2009; Kuiper *et al.*, 2009; Kassirer, 2010). Contemporary educational strategies for teaching the rational and analytic aspects of clinical decision-making are based upon principles of adult learning and integrate innovative methods, such as problem–based learning (Imanieh *et al.*, 2014; Jin and Bridges, 2014) and case study (Carr, 2015; Wadowski *et al.*, 2015), to support competence development in this area. Decision-making education is normally in a monoprofessional learning context and is focused at the level of the individual. Emphasis is placed on the rational model and the training of individual analytic thinking processes to solve clinical problems. Traditionally, little emphasis in undergraduate education has been given to decision-making in healthcare teams in collaboration with other health professionals, although this is an increasingly significant aspect of contemporary clinical practice.

The interprofessional education and collaboration movement in healthcare is, however, highlighting the fact that not only should healthcare professionals be educated and socialised within their chosen profession, but that today's graduates should also be emerging aware of the roles and responsibilities of other professions and have the ability to collaborate effectively in inter-professional healthcare teams (WHO, 2005a; Reeves *et al.*, 2008, 2010; Bals, 2009; Zwarenstein, Goldman and Reeves, 2009; Alscher *et al.*, 2010; CIHC, 2010; Frenk *et al.*, 2010; Thistlethwaite, Moran and WHO, 2010; IEC, 2011; Nisbet *et al.*, 2011; Tashiro *et al.*, 2011; Abu-Rish *et al.*, 2012). Interprofessional collaboration has been defined as: 'the process of developing and maintaining effective interprofessional working relationships with learners, practitioners, patients/clients/families and communities to enable optimal health outcomes' (CIHC, 2010, p. 8).

The *Framework for Action in Interprofessional Education and Collaborative Practice* promotes interprofessional education as a key strategy to enhance quality patient care outcomes by preparing a 'collaborative practice-ready health work-force' (WHO, 2010, p. 10). The ability of individual health professionals (those being dieticians, doctors, laboratory professionals, midwives, nurses, occupa-tional therapists, pharmacists, physiotherapists, radiographers, social workers, speech language therapists and so forth) to collaborate effectively within con-temporary healthcare teams is becoming a core aspect of modern professional practice.

European organisations, such as the UK Centre for the Advancement of Interprofessional Education (CAIPE) and the European Interprofessional Practice and Education Network (EIPEN) are active in developing and sharing resources for interprofessional education to support collaborative working relationships in healthcare. However, North American associations have led the way in the development of competency frameworks to guide collabo-rative interprofessional practice, where, due to the regulatory environment of the health professions, competency-based education and practice standards are already well established. The interprofessional competency domains in the Interprofessional Education Collaborative (IEC) framework from the US are as follows: values/ethics for interprofessional practice, roles/responsibilities, interprofessional communication, teams and teamwork (IEC, 2011, pp. 15–16). The Canadian Interprofessional Health Collaborative (CIHC) competency do-mains are: interprofessional communication, patient/client/family/community-centred care, role clarification, team functioning, collaborative leadership and interprofessional conflict resolution (CIHC, 2010, p. 9). The competencies identified in these frameworks are intended to build upon discipline-specific competencies from individual health professions (IEC, 2011, p. i). This can be seen in action with an example from the medical profession. One of the seven physician competency domains in *The CanMEDS 2005 Physician Competency Framework* is 'Collaborator': 'As *Collaborators* [sic], physicians effectively work within a healthcare team to achieve optimal care' (Frank, 2005, p. 15). Such competency-based frameworks highlight the need for today's health profes-sionals to be prepared with both the discipline-specific and interprofessional competencies required for their professional practice. The domains communi-cation, teamwork and role clarification are common to both interprofessional competency frameworks cited. Communication skills, teamwork abilities and understanding other team members' professional roles are also key factors that form the basis of being able to participate actively and thoughtfully in decision-making processes in healthcare teams.

Evolving models of decision–making in healthcare

Nevertheless, effective collaboration in decision–making processes at the organisational level can be inhibited by traditional hierarchies – where healthcare teams are also divided into professional silos – with their typically top-down structures (Sutton, 2009, p. 450). The problems this creates for effective collaborative working relationships in contemporary clinical practice are twofold. Particularly in the complex clinical environments with the fluctuating risk patterns of many Western health systems today, traditional hierarchical structures are no longer always appropriate for effective decision–making and can place undue burden on single individuals. Second, from the patient perspective, traditional hierarchies are no longer always appropriate for effective decision–making in healthcare, as more patients want to play an active role in decisions about their care (and should be doing so for their own benefit and safety). In *How Doctors Think* Groopman (2007) signals the importance of this when he says: 'Doctors desperately need patients and their families and friends to help them think. Without their help, physicians are denied key clues to what is really wrong' (Groopman, 2007, pp. 7–8). For such reasons, a gradual breakdown of hierarchical structures in healthcare is taking place (Witz, 1992, pp. 53–4) and this is being reflected in the emergence of new decision–making models in response to environmental need.

'Shared decision–making' is one such example. This inclusive partnership approach to decision–making is hierarchically a flatter structure, where the doctor shares decision–making power with the patient. It has its roots in the concepts of informed choice and consumer empowerment (Edwards and Elwyn, 2009, p. 4). Charles, Gafni and Whelan (1997) proposed the following principles for shared decision–making, which have found wide acceptance:

> Shared decision–making involves at least two participants – the physician and patient. Both parties (physicians and patients) take steps to participate in the process of treatment decision–making. Information sharing is a prerequisite to shared decision–making. A treatment decision is made and both parties agree on the decision.
>
> (Charles *et al.*, 1997, pp. 685–8)

Although this model is based on a physician–patient dyad, it does recognise the potential for a triad to be formed, where relatives or a friend may be included in decision–making processes (Charles *et al.*, 1997, p. 685) and it is also acknowledged that 'several physicians often participate in this process' (Charles *et al.*, 1997, p. 685) in complex care. The development of the shared decision–making model has been a significant step forward in improving the quality of decisions and patient safety in healthcare by integrating the patient's perspective into decision–making processes.

Collaborative decision–making – a hybrid model for healthcare

However, the primary limitation of the shared decision–making model is its physician–centric nature. This reaches its limits in complex care situations, particularly for patients with long–term chronic conditions or disability cared for by interprofessional teams. Early signs of a new decision–making model have appeared in recent literature. This is a hybrid entity, where the shared decision–making model has been widened beyond the physician–patient dyad to actively include other health professional groups by integrating the principles of interprofessional collaboration. Examples include a primary care setting in Canada (Légaré *et al.*, 2008) and a mental health setting in Australia (Chong, Aslani and Chen, 2013). The authors recognise this emergent hybrid development as a new decision–making model in healthcare and have termed it 'collaborative decision–making' (CDM), which is understood to be a normative synthesis of current best practice models in decision–making and collaborative interprofessional practice in healthcare (see Box 4.1).

Box 4.1   Collaborative decision–making – a hybrid model for healthcare

Interprofessional collaboration	**Shared decision–making**
The process of developing and maintaining effective interprofessional working relationships with learners, practitioners, patients/clients/ families and communities to enable optimal health outcomes (CIHC 2010, p. 8).	Involves at least two participants – the physician and the patient. Both parties take steps to participate in the process of treatment decision–making. Information sharing is a prerequisite to shared decision–making. A treatment decision is made and both parties agree on the decision (Charles *et al.* 1997, pp. 685–8).

Collaborative decision–making (definition)

The process by which interprofessional teams effectively work together in partnership with the patient/family in the process of decision–making in chronic and/or complex care situations and come to agreements that enable optimal health outcomes to be achieved with available resources.

CDM in itself is not an entirely new concept. It is used in emergency and disaster management to promote effective and coordinated consensus-based decisions by multiple agencies and has been defined as the 'combination and utilization of resources and management tools by several entities to achieve a common goal' (Kapucu and Garayev, 2011, p. 366). The CDM model itself originated in the aviation industry:

> There are two central tenants [*sic*]to CDM; that better information will lead to better decision–making, and tools and procedures need to be in place to enable air navigation service providers and the flight operators to more easily respond to changing conditions. By sharing information, values and preferences, stakeholders learn from each other and build a common pool of knowledge.
>
> (Federal Aviation Association, 2015)

CDM is a complex phenomenon which aims at reaching decisions amenable to all stakeholders, even when there are varying objectives or even conflicting interests. This is of particular relevance in complex patient care situations involving interprofessional healthcare teams where there may be professionally divergent goals, priorities and values (Renn, Klinke and van Asselt, 2011, p. 235), despite a shared general aim to provide quality patient care.

CDM has significant advantages for healthcare teams. It can harness team intelligence in a phenomenon known as 'distributed cognition' (Hutchins, 1996, p. 176; Gordon, Mendenhall and O'Connor, 2013, pp. 10–11), enabling health professionals to actively harness their combined knowledge bases and perspectives in decision–making, resulting in process gains for the benefit of the patient. This has significant potential to improve the timeliness and quality of decisions in healthcare. When decision–making is approached as a collaborative process between the patient/family and members of the interprofessional healthcare team, working together and sharing information effectively, then not only is patient safety actively promoted by enabling checking for error, but also positive synergies from combined knowledge bases and diverse perspectives are enabled. This results potentially in novel patient–centred solutions (Raiffa, Richardson and Metcalfe, 2002, pp. 17–18; Kahneman, 2011, pp. 417–18). This new hybrid entity, the CDM model in healthcare, has emerged in response to needs in the current practice environment and can be a valuable tool when used by healthcare teams for decision–making in partnership with patients/families to address chronic and/or complex health needs. It can support interprofessional teams to achieve optimal patient care outcomes in the dynamic health systems typifying clinical settings today.

Impact of dynamic health systems on cognitive processes

Despite the potential advantages of the CDM model in chronic and/or complex care applications, decision–making processes in healthcare do not often take place under ideal conditions, but in dynamic rapidly changing healthcare settings. This creates other challenges. Current healthcare environments are characterised by complexity, ambiguity and, increasingly, by workforce and resource constraints. Such dynamic environments make decision-making per se more difficult (Hodgkinson and Starbuck, 2008, p. 17; Kahneman, 2011, p. 341). First, complexity makes decisions difficult because the chain of events between cause and effect is hard to identify and quantify among a range of explanations and adverse effects (Renn *et al.*, 2011, p. 234). Second, ambiguity makes decisions more difficult because there are different legitimate viewpoints and values from which a decision can be evaluated and, therefore, not only divergent or contesting perspectives on the key issues (or problems or risks), but also on the ways to assess relevance and meaning and to determine action. Professionally divergent goals, priorities and values are, for example, a cause of ambiguity in the healthcare environment (Renn *et al.*, 2011, p. 235). Third, resource constraints can make decisions difficult (not to mention problematic to implement) regardless of whether the constraints are in the form of time, manpower, material goods or otherwise. Having to make choices and decisions in dynamic and complex healthcare systems is a significant cognitive challenge for health professionals.

Uncertainty created by critical or high-stake issues (for example, a rapidly deteriorating patient) adds further to the cognitive challenge, over and above the factors of complexity, ambiguity and resource constraints (Raiffa *et al.*, 2002, p. 38; Kapucu and Garayev, 2011, p. 368), and all these factors impact negatively on the final decision-making quality (Kahneman, 2011, p. 14). Human limitations in cognitive processing ability lead to the (mostly unconscious) inclination to reduce variables and make short cuts in thinking to prevent cognitive overload (Hammond, Keeney and Raiffa, 1998; Elstein and Schwarz, 2002, p. 732; Arocha, Wang and Patel, 2005, p. 154). Kahneman, Slovic and Tversky (1982, p. 48) showed in a series of studies that:

> in making predictions and judgments under uncertainty, people do not appear to follow the calculus of chance or statistical theory of prediction. Instead, they rely on a limited number of heuristics which sometimes yield reasonable judgments and sometime lead to severe and systematic error.

When confronted with complexity, ambiguity, resources constraints and uncertainty in rapidly changing situations in a dynamic healthcare environment, health professionals are vulnerable to making inadvertent errors of judgement due to cognitive overload. This can lead to patient harm.

Fallible humans and systems failures

Decision-making research has shown that there are, in fact, a number of barriers to making rational judgements in complex and dynamic environments such as healthcare. Novices are especially vulnerable in complex environments, because of their inexperience (Dreyfus and Dreyfus, 1980). They need instructional feedback on how to make sense of a situation or context within a 'decision frame' (Tversky and Kahneman, 1981; Gong *et al.*, 2013) in their process of decision-making competence development. However, even experienced decision-makers are subject to the qualitative shortcomings of human decision-making (heuristics of judgement) that produces various kinds of mental lapses leading to bias, over-confidence and other hidden traps (Hammond *et al.*, 1998; Raiffa *et al.*, 2002, pp. 34–6). In addition, wider dimensions, such as professional norms (Tamuz and Lewis, 2008, p. 162), social power structures (Bandura, 1986, p. 29) and organisational environment, can limit information exchange and, thus, rationality in decision-making (Rojot, 2008, p. 149). Furthermore, when faced with uncertainty in complex environments, there is a tendency for a type of 'group think' to develop, where people anchor onto the judgements of others when making up their own mind during the decision-making process (Raiffa *et al.*, 2002, p. 38; Larrick, 2007). It is clear that a multiplicity of factors can hinder rational thinking processes and have a negative influence on the quality of decision-making at the best of times. Simply said, humans are error prone and the risk for health professionals to make mistakes is heightened due to the complex, dynamic environments in which they practise.

Hammond makes a strong case for the fact that, due to the element of 'irreducible uncertainty' in decision-making, mistakes are inevitable sooner or later (Hammond, 2000, p. 5). In healthcare, this results in adverse events, such as medication errors (Bates *et al.*, 1995), hospital-acquired infections (Haller *et al.*, 2014; Herzig *et al.*, 2014), wrong site surgery (Ambe, Sommer and Zirngibl, 2015; Pauli *et al.*, 2015) and error in medical diagnosis and treatment (Groopman, 2007, pp. 7–8; Graber, 2013). However, adverse events causing patient harm in complex systems such as healthcare organisations are not only a result of individual fallibility. Factors originating at different levels of the system also compromise patient safety due to latent failures and poor oversight, which creates an environment for unsafe processes (Jha *et al.*, 2010, p. 43). To date, evidence is mainly from hospital settings in developed nations and evidence in primary care systems and from transitioning and undeveloped nations is less robust (Jha *et al.*, 2010, p. 43). System-level failures resulting in medical error for hospital-level care in developed nations include: manpower problems, such as short staffing (Buchan and Aiken, 2008; Wise, 2014); production pressure creating heavy workloads (Kirby and Hurst, 2014; Nishimura *et al.*, 2014); 'traditions', such as extended duration shifts causing stress and fatigue issues (Barger *et al.*, 2006; Griffiths *et al.*, 2014); and poor organisational safety culture (Mulcahy, 2014; Speck *et al.*, 2014). In addition, an unknown number of errors go unreported (Henneman, 2007) and even when employees voice their concerns, organisations, in turn, can fail to respond and learn (WHO, 2005b; Jones and Kelly, 2014). Factors at both an individual and system level contribute to poor decision-making outcomes leading to adverse events and, therefore, appropriate decision-making models are essential tools for health professionals to be able to practise safely. The CDM model in healthcare has its part to play in optimising decision-making processes and ensuring safe outcomes for those patients with chronic and/or complex care needs being cared for in today's dynamic, rapidly changing health systems.

Conclusion

The ability to collaborate effectively in contemporary interprofessional health-care teams is a core aspect of modern professional practice. Communication skills, teamwork abilities and understanding other team members' professional roles and responsibilities are key factors that form the basis of being able to participate actively and thoughtfully in CDM processes. Having to make choices and decisions in dynamic and complex healthcare systems is a significant cognitive challenge. When confronted with uncertainty in rapidly changing situations in a dynamic healthcare environment, health professionals are vulnerable to making errors of judgement, which can lead to patient harm. Factors at both an individual and system level contribute to adverse outcomes and medical error. A multiplicity of factors can have a negative influence on decision quality and the conscious awareness of common barriers to rationality is the best defence against this. The development of the shared decision-making model was a significant step forward in improving quality and safety in health-care by integrating the patient's perspective into decision-making processes. A new model of CDM in healthcare has emerged as a synthesis of current best practice models in shared decision-making and interprofessional practice. The CDM model enables richer decision-making processes for complex patient care to achieve optimal health outcomes in dynamic health systems.

Authors' note

The authors' acknowledge that in writing this chapter their lens has been focused primarily on hospital-level care in developed Western nations and they have drawn on evidence almost exclusively from North America and Western Europe.

References

Abu-Rish, E., Kim, S., Choe, L., Varpio, L., Malik, E., White, A.A. *et al.*, 2012. Current trends in interprofessional education of health sciences students: a literature review. *Journal of Interprofessional Care*, 26(6), pp. 444–51.

Alscher, M.D., Büscher, A., Dielmann, G., Hopfeld, M., Höppner, H., Igl, G. *et al.*, 2010. *Memorandum Kooperation der Gesundheitsberufe. Qualität und Sicherung der Gesundheitsversorgung von morgen.* [pdf] Stuttgart: Robert Bosch Stiftung. Available through: <www.bosch-stiftung.de/content/language1/downloads/Memorandum_ Kooperation_der_Gesundheitsberufe.pdf> [accessed 9 July 2015].

Ambe, P.C., Sommer, B. and Zirngibl, H., 2015. Wrong site surgery: incidence, risk factors and prevention. *Der Chirurg* [Epub ahead of print] Published 13 February

2015. Available through: <http://link.springer.com/article/10.1007%2Fs00104-014-2983-8> [accessed 9 July 2015]. doi: 10. 1007/s00104-014-2983-8.

Arocha, J.F., Wang, D. and Patel V.L., 2005. Identifying reasoning strategies in medical decision making: a methodological guide. *Journal of Biomedical Informatics*, April, 38(2), pp. 154–71.

Bals, T., 2009. *Wege zur Ausbildungsqualität: Stand und Perspektiven in den Gesundheits fachberufen.* Paderborn: Eusl-Verlag.

Bandura, A., 1986. *Social foundations of thought and action: a social cognitive theory.* Englewood Cliffs, NJ: Prentice Hall.

Barger, L.K., Ayas, N.T., Cade, B.E., Cronin, J.W., Rosner, B., Speizer, F.E. and Czeisler, C.A., 2006. Impact of extended-duration shifts on medical errors, adverse events and attentional failures. *PLoS Medicine*, 3(12), p.e487.

Bates, D.W., Cullen, D.J., Laird, N., Peterson, L.A., Small, S.D., Servi, D. *et al.*, 1995. Incidence of adverse drug events and potential adverse drug events. Implications for prevention. *Journal of the American Medical Association*, 274(1), pp. 29–34.

Buchan, J. and Aiken, L., 2008. Solving nursing shortages: a common priority. *Journal of Clinical Nursing*, 17(24), pp. 3262–8.

Carr, K.C., 2015. Using the unfolding case study in midwifery education. *Journal of Midwifery and Women's Health*, [Epub ahead of print] Published 8 May 2015. Available through: <http://onlinelibrary.wiley.com/doi/10.1111/jmwh.12293/abstract;jsessionid=83765ABCAF72BF21591282CF42001D90.f04t02> [accessed 9 July 2015].

Charles, C., Gafni, A. and Whelan, T., 1997. Shared decision-making in the medical encounter: what does it mean? (or it takes at least two to tango). *Social Science and Medicine*, 44(5), pp. 681–92.

Chong, W.W., Aslani, P. and Chen, T., 2013. Shared decision-making and inter-professional collaboration in mental healthcare: a qualitative study exploring perceptions of barriers and facilitators. *Journal of Interprofessional Care*, 27(5), pp. 373–9.

CIHC: Canadian Interprofessional Health Collaborative, 2010. *A national interprofessional competency framework.* [pdf] Vancouver BC: Canadian Interprofessional Health Collaborative. Available through: <http://www.cihc.ca/files/CIHC_IPCompetencies_Feb1210.pdf> [accessed 9 July 2015].

Dreyfus, S.E. and Dreyfus, H.L., 1980. *A five-stage model of the mental activities involved in directed skill acquisition.* Report No: ORC 80-2. University of Berkley, CA: Operations Research Center, pp. 1–18.

Edwards, A. and Elwyn, G. eds., 2009. *Shared decision-making in health care. Achieving evidence-based patient choice.* 2nd ed. Oxford and New York: Oxford University Press.

Elstein, A.S. and Schwarz, A., 2002. Clinical problem solving and diagnostic decision making: a selective review of the cognitive literature. *British Medical Journal*, 324(7339), pp. 729–32.

Federal Aviation Association, 2015. *CDM Home. Improving air traffic management together.* Available through: <http://cdm.fly.faa.gov/> [accessed 9 July 2015].

Frank, J.R. ed., 2005. *The CanMEDS 2005 Physician competency framework. Better standards. Better physicians. Better care.* Ottawa, ON: The Royal College of Physicians and Surgeons Canada. Available through: <www.royalcollege.ca/portal/page/portal/rc/common/documents/canmeds/resources/publications/framework_full_e.pdf> [accessed 9 July 2015].

Frenk, J., Chen, L., Bhutta, Z.A., Cohen, J., Crisp, N., Evans, T. *et al.*, 2010. Health professionals for a new century: transforming education to strengthen health systems in an interdependent world. *Lancet*, 376(9756), pp. 1923–58.

Gong, J., Zhang, Y., Huang, Y., Feng, J. and Zhang, W., 2013. The framing effects in medical decision-making: a review of the literature. *Psychology, Health and Medicine*, 18(6), pp. 645–53.

Gordon, S., Mendenhall, P. and O'Connor, B., 2013. *Beyond the checklist. What else health care can learn from aviation teamwork and safety.* Ithaca, NY and London: ILP Press.

Graber, M.L., 2013. The incidence of diagnostic error in medicine. *BMJ Quality and Safety*, 22(Suppl. 2), pp. ii21–ii27.

Griffiths, P., Dall'Ora, C., Simon, M., Ball, J., Lindqvist, R., Rafferty, A. *et al.*, 2014. Nurses' shift length and overtime working in 12 European countries: the association with perceived quality of care and patient safety. *Medical Care*, 52(11), pp. 975–81.

Groopman, J., 2007. *How doctors think.* Boston, MA: Houghton Mifflin Company.

Haller, C., Eckmanns, T., Benzler, J., Tolksdorf, K., Claus, H., Gilsdorf, A. and Sin, M., 2014. Results from the first 12 months of the national surveillance of healthcare associated outbreaks in Germany, 2011/2012. *PLoS one*, 9(5), p.e98100. Available online: <http://journals.plos.org/plosone/article?id=10.1371/journal.pone.0098100> [accessed 9 July 2015].

Hammond, J.S., Keeney, R.L. and Raiffa, H., 1998. The hidden traps in decision making. *Harvard Business Review*, 76(5), pp. 47–8, 50, 52.

Hammond, K., 2000. *Human judgment and social policy: irreducible uncertainty, inevitable error, unavoidable justice.* Oxford and London: Oxford University Press.

Hendrick, P., Bond, C., Duncan, E. and Hale, L., 2009. Clinical reasoning in musculoskeletal practice: students' conceptualizations. *Physical Therapy*, 89(5), pp. 430–42.

Henneman, E.A., 2007. Unreported errors in the intensive care unit: a case study of the way we work. *Critical Care Nurse*, 27(5), pp. 27–34.

Herzig, C.T., Reagan, J., Pogorzelska-Maziarz, M., Srinath, D. and Stone, P., 2014. State-mandated reporting of health care-associated infections in the United States: trends over time. *American Journal of Medical Quality*, [Epub ahead of print] Published 20 June 2014. Available through: <http://ajm.sagepub.com/content/early/2014/06/20/1062860614540200.long> [accessed 9 July 2015]. doi: 10.1177/10628606 14540200.

Hicks, R.B., Geist, M.J. and House, M.J., 2013. SAFETY: an integrated clinical reasoning and reflection framework for undergraduate nursing students. *Journal of Nursing Education*, 52(1), pp. 59–62.

Hodgkinson, G. and Starbuck, W. eds., 2008. *The Oxford handbook of organizational decision making.* Oxford and New York: Oxford University Press.

Hutchins, E., 1996. *Cognition in the wild.* Cambridge, MA: MIT Press.

IEC: Interprofessional Education Collaborative Expert Panel, 2011. *Core competencies for interprofessional collaborative practice: Report of an expert panel.* [pdf] Washington, DC: Interprofessional Education Collaborative. Available through: <www.aacn.nche.edu/education-resources/ipecreport.pdf> [accessed 9 July 2015].

Imanieh, M.H., Dehghani, S.M., Sobhani, A.R. and Haghighat, M., 2014. Evaluation of problem-based learning in medical students' education. *Journal of Advances in Medical Education and Professionalism*, 2(1), pp. 1–5.

Jha, A.K., Prasopa-Plaizier, N., Larizgoitia, I., Bates, D., and Research Priority Setting Working Group of the WHO World Alliance for Patient Safety, 2010. Patient safety research: an overview of the global evidence. *Quality and Safety in Health Care*, 19(1), pp. 42–7.

Jin, J. and Bridges, S.M., 2014. Educational technologies in problem-based learning in health sciences education: a systematic review. *Journal of Medical Internet Research*, 16(12), p. e251.

Jones, A. and Kelly, D., 2014. Deafening silence? Time to reconsider whether organisations are silent or deaf when things go wrong. *BMJ Quality and Safety*, 23(9), pp. 709–13.

Kahneman, D., 2011. *Thinking fast and slow*. London: Penguin Books.

Kahneman, D., Slovic, P. and Tversky, A., 1982. *Judgment under uncertainty: heuristics and biases*. Cambridge: Cambridge University Press.

Kapucu, N. and Garayev, V., 2011. Collaborative decision-making in emergency and disaster management. *International Journal of Public Administration*, 34, pp. 366–75.

Kassirer, J.P., 2010. Teaching clinical reasoning: case-based and coached. *Academic Medicine: Journal of the Association of American Medical Colleges*, 85(7), pp. 1118–24.

Kirby, E. and Hurst, K., 2014. Using a complex audit tool to measure workload, staffing and quality in district nursing. *British Journal of Community Nursing*, 19(5), pp. 219–23.

Kuiper, R., Pesut, D. and Kautz, D., 2009. Promoting the self-regulation of clinical reasoning skills in nursing students. *The Open Nursing Journal*, 3, pp. 76–85.

Larrick, R., 2007. Debiasing. In: D. Koehler and N. Harvey, eds. *Blackwell handbook of judgment and decision making*. [e-book]. Malden, MA: Blackwell Publishing.

Légaré, F., Stacey, D., Graham, I.D., Elwyn, G., Pluye, P., Gagnon, M.P. *et al.*, 2008. Advancing theories, models and measurement for an interprofessional approach to shared decision making in primary care: a study protocol. *BMC Health Services Research*, 8(2), pp. 1–8.

Mulcahy, L., 2014. The market for precedent: shifting visions of the role of clinical negligence claims and trials. *Medical Law Review*, 22 (2), pp. 274–90.

Neistadt, M.E. and Atkins, A., 1996. Analysis of the orthopedic content in an occupational therapy curriculum from a clinical reasoning perspective. *American Journal of Occupational Therapy*, 50(8), pp. 669–75.

Nisbet, G., Lee, A., Kumar, K., Thistlethwaite, J. and Dunston, R., 2011. *Interprofessional health education: a literature review. Overview of international and Australian developments in interprofessional health education (IPE)*. [pdf]. Sydney, Australia: Centre for Research in Learning and Change University of Technology. Available through: <www.health.wa.gov.au/wactn/docs/IPEAUSlitreview2011.pdf> [accessed 9 July 2015].

Nishimuru, K., Nakamura, F., Takegami, M., Fukuhara, S., Nakagawara, J., Ogasawara, K. *et al.*, 2014. Cross-sectional survey of workload and burnout among Japanese physicians working in stroke care: the nationwide survey of acute stroke care capacity for proper designation of comprehensive stroke center in Japan (J-ASPECT) study. *Circulation, Cardiovascular Quality and Outcomes*, 7(3), pp. 414–22.

Pauli, D.E., Mazzia, L.M., Neily, J., Mills, P.D., Turner, J.R., Gunnar, W. and Hemphill, R., 2015. Errors upstream and downstream to the universal protocol associated with wrong surgery events in the Veterans Health Administration. *American Journal of Surgery*, 210(1), pp. 6–13.

Raiffa, H., Richardson, J. and Metcalfe, D., 2002. *Negotiation analysis: the science and art of collaborative decision making.* Cambridge, MA: Belknap.

Reeves, S., Zwarenstein, M., Goldman, J., Barr, H., Freeth, D., Hammick, M. and Koppel, I., 2008. Interprofessional education: effects on professional practice and health care outcomes. *Cochrane Database of Systematic Reviews,* [online] 23(1), CD002213. Available through: <http://onlinelibrary.wiley.com/doi/10.1002/14651858.CD002213.pub2/full> [accessed on 9 July 2015].

Renn, O., Klinke, A. and van Asselt, M., 2011. Coping with complexity, uncertainty and ambiguity in risk governance: a synthesis. *Ambio*, 40(2), pp. 231–46.

Rojot, J., 2008. Culture and decision making. In: G. Hodgkinson and W. Starbuck, eds. *The Oxford handbook of organizational decision making.* Oxford and New York: Oxford University Press. Ch. 7.

Speck, R.M., Foster, J.J., Mulhern, V.A., Burke, S.V., Sullivan, P.G. and Fleisher, L.A., 2014. Development of a professionalism committee approach to address unprofessional medical staff behavior at an academic medical center. *Joint Commission Journal on Quality and Safety*, 40(4), pp. 161–7.

Sutton, G., 2009. Evaluating multidisciplinary health care teams: taking the crisis out of CRM. *Australian Health Review*, 33(3), pp. 445–52.

Tamuz, M. and Lewis, E., 2008. Facing the threat of disaster: decision making when the stakes are high. In: G. Hodgkinson and W. Starbuck, eds., *The Oxford handbook of organizational decision making.* Oxford and New York: Oxford University Press, Ch. 8.

Tashiro, J., Byrne, C., Kitchen, L., Vogel, E. and Bianco, C., 2011. The development of competencies in interprofessional healthcare for use in health sciences educational programmes. *Journal of Research in Interprofessional Practice and Education*, 2(1), pp. 63–82. Available through: <www.jripe.org/index.php/journal/article/view/64/46> [accessed 9 July 2015].

Thistlethwaite, J., Moran, M. and WHO: World Health Organization Study Group on Interprofessional Education and Collaborative Practice, 2010. Learning outcomes for international education (IPE): literature review and synthesis. *Journal of Interprofessional Care*, 24(5), pp. 503–13.

Tversky, A. and Kahneman, D., 1981. The framing of decisions and the psychology of choice. *Science*, 211(4481), pp. 4538.

Wadowski, P.P., Steinlechner, B., Schiferer, A. and Löffler-Stastka, H., 2015. From clinical reasoning to effective clinical decision-making – new training methods. *Frontiers in Psychology*, 21 April, 6, p. 473.

WHO: World Health Organization, 2005a. *Preparing a health care workforce for the 21st century: the challenge of chronic conditions.* [pdf] Geneva, Switzerland: World Health Organization. Available through: <www.who.int/chp/knowledge/publications/workforce_report.pdf?ua=1> [accessed 9 July 2015].

WHO: World Health Organization, World Alliance for Patient Safety, 2005b. *WHO Draft guidelines for adverse event reporting and learning systems. From information to action.* [pdf] Geneva, Switzerland: World Health Organization. Available through: <http://osp.od.nih.gov/sites/default/files/resources/Reporting_Guidelines.pdf> [accessed 9 July 2015].

WHO: World Health Organization, 2010. *Framework for action on interprofessional education and collaborative practice.* [pdf] Geneva, Switzerland: World Health Organization. Available through: <http://whqlibdoc.who.int/hq/2010/WHO_HRH_HPN_10.3_eng.pdf?ua=1> [accessed 9 July 2015].

Wise, J., 2014. Stroke care audit shows major staff shortages. *British Medical Journal*, 349, p. g7407.

Witz, A., 1992. *Professions and patriarchy*. London: Routledge.

Zwarenstein, M., Goldman, J. and Reeves, S., 2009. Interprofessional collaboration: effects of practice-based interventions on professional practice and healthcare outcomes. *Cochrane Database of Systematic Reviews*, [online] 8(3), p. CD000072. Available through: <http://onlinelibrary.wiley.com/doi/10.1002/14651858.CD000072.pub2/full> [accessed on 9 July 2015]. doi: 10.1002/14651858.CD000072.pub2.

5 The Regensburg Model ('Pain Care Manager')

An integrated interprofessional pain curriculum for healthcare professionals in German-speaking countries

Kirstin Fragemann, Nicole Lindenberg, Bernhard M. Graf and Christoph H. R. Wiese

Background and definition of the problem

Why does pain present a major challenge to healthcare providers?

The incidence of pain in the German and European population demonstrates that the effective treatment of pain is still a big challenge for healthcare professionals (Breivik *et al.*, 2006; van den Beuken *et al.*, 2007; Deandrea, 2008; Burke and Shorten, 2009; Maier *et al.*, 2010). The efficient treatment of pain is a complex phenomenon requiring both the initiative of the multi-disciplinary healthcare team and organisational structures in healthcare institutions (Fragemann *et al.*, 2012).

Healthcare professionals need to be able to manage pain competently and effectively. A variety of reviews of pain knowledge among healthcare professionals report low education and insufficient qualifications (Bhamb *et al.*, 2006; Lin *et al.*, 2008; Pflughaupt *et al.*, 2010; Johnson, Collett and Castro-Lopes, 2013). The lack of knowledge in areas of pain medicine and misbeliefs about opioids carry the greatest risk for under- or overmedication of pain, consequently affecting patients' quality of life (Irajpour, 2006; Hunter *et al.*, 2008; Carr and Watt-Watson, 2012; Watt-Watson, Siddall and Carr, 2012). Apart from theoretical knowledge, specific collaborative competencies related to pain management are minimal for many healthcare professionals (Watt-Watson *et al.*, 2004; Irajpour, 2006; Watt-Watson *et al.*, 2012). Until recently, healthcare professionals have often maintained competitive, tense or dependent relationships, which result from a lack of precise definitions and concepts regarding their responsibilities within a complex clinical environment (Fragemann *et al.*, 2012).

Therefore, pain education must involve healthcare professionals at all levels to improve practical skills and clinical outcomes (Irajpour, 2006; Carr and Watt-Watson, 2012; Johnson *et al.*, 2013). One medical professional alone cannot overcome the complex challenge of providing skilled pain management in chronic pain patients (Carr and Watt-Watson, 2012; Watt-Watson *et al.*, 2012).

Pain education is essential for all healthcare professionals –
current education policies and initiatives in Europe

Although pain education has been identified as a strategy to improve ineffective pain management practices, recent evidence demonstrates the continuing lack of pain education in health science curricula (Watt-Watson *et al.*, 2004, 2012; Briggs, Carr and Whittaker, 2011; Mundipharma, 2013; Briggs, 2014). In fact, curriculum guidelines have been created by national and international pain societies to encourage the integration of pain education in the regular medical school curricula. The International Association for the Study of Pain (IASP) published the first edition of a Core Curriculum for Professional Education in Pain (1991) more than 20 years ago (IASP, 2012). The IASP provided special core curricula for the different healthcare professions (e.g. psychologists and physiotherapists) to ensure general access to pain education for health professionals (IASP, 2015). However, these current efforts may not be enough to eliminate insufficient pain control (Briggs *et al.*, 2011; Mundipharma, 2013; Briggs, 2014). Despite advances in curriculum development, a survey of UK universities, which was published in 2011, revealed an average of only 12 hours of undergraduate pain education during the whole period of study (Briggs *et al.*, 2011). A survey of 242 undergraduate medical schools in Europe also explored a limited average number of hours concerning pain-related subjects (Mundipharma, 2013). On average, pain education accounted for 0.2 per cent of the undergraduate medical schools teaching (Mundipharma, 2013).

According to the German Pain Association, approximately half of the 36 medical schools extant in Germany are teaching pain management (German Pain Association, 2012). However, the recent introduction of amendments to the medical licensure laws has led to the introduction of pain medicine as a specific topic in the medical curriculum, and this must be implemented by all faculties by 2016 (Bredanger *et al.*, 2008; German Pain Association, 2012; Fragemann and Wiese, 2014; The Medical Association of North Rhine (ÄkNo), 2014).

Furthermore, there are different approaches to post-licensure programmes at the national level. Due to the absence of regulations, there is variation and relatively uncontrolled growth in pain education for medical assistance occupations (Fragemann and Wiese, 2011, 2014). A piece of Internet-based research which was conducted in 2011 revealed the existence of more than 40 different pain education programmes for nurses in Austria, Germany and Switzerland. While these courses demonstrate a general consensus on learning objectives, there is a huge range of course titles and lengths, from 8–192 hours. A national committee of the German Nurses Association is currently attempting to unite the professional interests of German pain nurses (Fragemann and Wiese, 2011, 2014). However, physiotherapists, occupational healthcare therapists and pharmacists have no opportunity to choose a formal course programme that is legally regulated in Germany. The clinical subspecialisation 'Special pain therapy' is legally regulated by the German Medical Association, and only physicians are entitled to perform it. Psychologists in Germany can also complete a formal education in the special psychotherapeutic treatment of pain.

Better pain education in the undergraduate curriculum is important to ensure that young professionals entering clinical practice will be well trained in pain management. It is fundamental for post-licensure healthcare professionals to ensure a patient-centred collaboration and to improve existing barriers, such as poor interprofessional and interdisciplinary communication and traditional but obsolete mutual role expectations (Hunter *et al.*, 2008). Consequently, the IASP published a core curriculum on interprofessional pain education in 2012, mentioned previously (IASP, 2012). In 2014, the British Pain Society constituted national recommendations for universities on interprofessional pain education (Briggs, 2014). While English-speaking countries have gained some years of experience in supporting interprofessional education, in Germany, little effort has been made regarding interprofessional pain management for undergraduate students and post-licensure healthcare professionals. One national programme to enhance the efficacy of pain management in the field of further education is the Regensburg Model, which aims at developing an integrated interprofessional pain curriculum (Fragemann *et al.*, 2012; Fragemann and Wiese, 2014).

Interprofessional education in the context of clinical practice

Interprofessional education and collaborative practice to enhance the quality of care

Increasing demand shows us that the era of lone fighters among healthcare professionals is over. The move towards an interprofessional clinical environment is fraught with many hurdles, and we need learning strategies to support a closer collaboration among healthcare professionals (Pargeon and Hailey, 1999; Pollard, Sellman and Thomas, 2014).

Working as an interprofessional team means planning, managing and monitoring care, and communicating or coordinating care may result in more effective and safe patient outcomes (Gilbert, Yan and Hoffman, 2010; Watt–Watson *et al.*, 2012). Interprofessionality in healthcare systems across the world is a response to the growing fragmentation of clinical practices (D'Amour and Oandasan, 2005). Healthcare professionals undergo different types of vocational training at different levels of qualification, and each profession is socialised in a specific profession-immanent field of activity concerning ethos and role description. Against this background, healthcare professionals have different concepts of the patients' needs and the way in which to respond to complex care situations (D'Amour and Oandasan, 2005). The concept of interprofessionality in terms of a collaborative practice is described as the development of a cohesive practice between professionals from different healthcare professions and disciplines (D'Amour and Oandasan, 2005). Above all, this means that healthcare professionals enter into a process characterised by a targeted reflection on ways to practice and the provision of care determined by the shared perspectives of all team members involved in the patients' treatment (D'Amour and Oandasan, 2005). Developing and instilling interprofessional practice requires a deeper understanding of the key factors that influence both interprofessional practice and interprofessional education. A crucial prerequisite for effective collaboration in healthcare domains is the support of innovative learning approaches, which prepare healthcare professionals to participate effectively as members of interprofessional healthcare teams (Carr, 2003). There are numerous approaches towards interprofessional education internationally, and it is a great challenge to improve continuing medical education and collaborative practice (WHO, 1988; Carr and Watt-Watson, 2012). In addition to enhancing knowledge, interprofessional education aims to overcome negative professional stereotypes and to lay the foundation for shared decision-making (Carpenter, 1995; Watt-Watson *et al.*, 2004; D'Amour, 2005; D'Amour and Oandasan, 2005; Irajpour, 2006; Hammick *et al.*, 2007; Hunter *et al.*, 2008; Carr and Watt-Watson, 2012; Reeves *et al.*, 2013). Implementing interprofessional education may generate new ideas and attitudes to improve the departmental culture and collaborative teamwork (Dudley and Wiysonge, 2008). Improving the competencies of all team members through an interprofessional approach may also contribute to a reduced rate of clinical errors and better clinical outcomes (Dudley and Wiysonge, 2008).

Definitions and key elements of interprofessional working and learning approaches

Interprofessionalism can be described with a theoretical framework. D'Amour (2005) reviewed the scientific literature to describe certain aspects of interprofessionalism and collaboration. The author identified four main concepts strongly linked to interprofessional practice. The first concept is collaboration, which is a key factor connected to determinants such as 'sharing', 'partnership', 'power' and 'interdependence'. 'Sharing' plays a central role in numerous references. Consequently, collaboration depends on various elements, such as 'shared decision-making', 'shared healthcare philosophy', 'shared professional values' and 'shared clinical planning and intervention'. Furthermore, a collaborative approach requires the element of partnership, which is frequently characterised by a constructive and true relationship based on mutual respect and common working goals. Collaborative practice is also linked to the mutual dependence of professionals within a healthcare team. Working together in a close collaboration implies that each team member is necessary for the outcome. Finally, power seems crucial to a collaborative practice and it is expressed through the democratic interaction of the team members with various degrees of knowledge and clinical experience. It is also essential to utilise teamwork, which is the centre of collaborative and patient-centred care (D'Amour, 2005).

New learning approaches are necessary, which consistently promote collaborative skills, to achieve increased interprofessional collaboration. Interprofessional education has been defined as two or more professions learning with, from and about each other to improve collaborative practice and the quality of care (CAIPE, 2002; Gilbert *et al.*, 2010). Interprofessionality is often mistaken for multiprofessionality, which also involves different professions (Watt-Watson *et al.*, 2012). However, there are some important differences related to the learning approach and the clinical environment. Multiprofessional education involves different professions, but students learn simultaneously and usually with a minimal interaction or sharing of roles (Watt-Watson *et al.*, 2012). Consequently, interprofessional education requires more than learning together in a classroom. In fact, successful outcomes from an interprofessional teaching approach require interactive teaching elements that aim at enabling students to enter into open dialogue (Carr, 2003; Watt-Watson *et al.*, 2012).

Using interprofessional education to teach pain management: what effects can we expect?

Interprofessional education can be seen as an appropriate learning approach to overcome barriers between healthcare professionals, such as the elimination of prejudices and stereotypes (Carpenter, 1995; D'Amour and Oandasan, 2005; Strickland, Huskey and Brushwood, 2007). Interprofessional course programmes have been positively evaluated internationally regarding attitudes towards the acceptance of interprofessional education strategies and the readiness to work in collaborative ways with others (McFadyen *et al.*, 2005; Pollard and Miers, 2008; Hertweck *et al.*, 2012; Pollard *et al.*, 2014). In a number of studies, representatives from various professional fields in different groupings were involved: physicians, nurses, pharmacists, psychologists, physiotherapists and occupational healthcare therapists (Strickland *et al.*, 2007; Aziz, Chong Tek and Yen Yen, 2011). Because physicians and nurses are the largest group of healthcare workers, they have been the subjects of previous research within the framework of interprofessional education. However, pharmacists have become a more integral part of the healthcare team and must prepare for new ways of working. They collaborate with patients, their families and other healthcare providers in different healthcare settings. Consequently, pharmacists are increasingly becoming a focus in the context of interprofessional education (Strickland *et al.*, 2007).

The improvement of knowledge about pain and pain management within interprofessional education projects was given a positive assessment (Carr, 2003; Irajpour, 2006; Lin *et al.*, 2008; Watt-Watson *et al.*, 2012). With regard to the effects on clinical practice, research demonstrated changes in pain documentation and an increase of pain assessment (Irajpour, 2006). Other findings placed the focus on patients and suggested a positive impact on pain intensity and patient satisfaction (Carr, 2003; Irajpour, 2006; Lin *et al.*, 2008).

However, not a lot of published data exists concerning pain curricula for post-licensure students who have already gained clinical experience and a certain status within the team hierarchy. The majority of the programmes evaluated were held in the field of undergraduate seminars (Zwarenstein, Reeves and Perrier, 2005; Zwarenstein, Goldman and Reeves, 2009). There are hardly any concretely defined and standardised curricula on pain management in further education in the area of interprofessional learning approaches for graduated healthcare professionals (Fragemann and Wiese, 2011; Fragemann *et al.*, 2012).

Implementing an integrated interprofessional curriculum for healthcare professionals in German-speaking countries ('Pain Care Manager')

Curricular objectives

The identification of existing deficiencies in the provision of interprofessional perspectives on the treatment of pain has motivated the initiation of a cross-curricular project regarding pain management for post-licensure healthcare professionals. The structured dialogue on the subject of interprofessional education in pain management was a project shared between the Department of Anaesthesiology and the Centre for Education with a focus on nursing science. The curriculum was designed as a core curriculum to complement the curricula on pain management already extant in German-speaking countries which have been accredited or recognised by the national pain societies and the different professional associations. The existing medical guidelines and recommendations for further education in pain management were integrated into the interprofessional course concept for quality assurance and transparency with regard to dissemination and the use of the course contents. The purpose of the development of the pain curriculum was to enhance knowledge about pain mechanisms, pain assessment, principles of medical treatment and complementary therapies in the context of interprofessional perspectives on the management of patients suffering from acute, chronic or malignant pain conditions. Additionally, monoprofessional issues, which are crucial for pain management, have been integrated. The interprofessional education approach was designed to serve as a post-licensure model to promote an interactive dialogue and to simplify the communication between the different professions involved in the treatment process. The challenge was to respond to the needs of as many people as possible, because communication between different professional groups is often difficult as they have different vocabularies and mentalities. While the undergraduate curricula focus on knowledge about the roles of different professionals, the Regensburg Model, which is a post-licensure curriculum, involves clinical experiences with patients and the individual's role as part of a healthcare team.

Process of curriculum development

An expert panel led by a physician and nurse educator was established to foster interprofessionalism within the project team. The working group was composed of experts representing anaesthesiology and special pain therapy, psychology, pharmacology, nursing science and nursing education.

A six-step approach to curriculum development was used (Kern *et al.*, 1998) for the compilation of a concept:

1 identify the problem;
2 conduct a needs assessment;
3 set goals and objectives based on the needs identified;
4 select educational strategies to meet the goals;
5 implementation; and
6 evaluation.

A literature review on pain education for undergraduate and graduate pain curricula, both generally and particularly for German-speaking countries, was performed. We searched PubMed, EMBASE and Google Scholar in January 2011 and made the literature search again in January 2015 to update the educational requirements. Additionally, the working group conducted an Internet-based study in 2011 using Google to identify the existing range of courses related to pain management in Germany, Austria and Switzerland. In summary, this Internet-based research demonstrated that there is currently no culture of interprofessionalism regarding pain education in German-speaking countries.

The design of the curriculum is integrative, is used to specify the concept and is based on the (1) Core Curriculum 'Special Pain Therapy' (post-licensure programme) (German Medical Association), (2) Integrated Pain Curriculum for Nurses (pre-licensure and post-licensure nurse education programme) (German Pain Association), (3) Core Curriculum for Professional Education in Pain (IASP Third Edition) and (4) Curriculum on Pain for Schools of Occupational Therapy and Physical Therapy (IASP, 2012).

The curriculum structure and implementation was aligned with the recommendations from Watt–Watson, Siddall and Carr (2012), who described the key elements of an interprofessional pain curriculum as follows:

• common basis for different professions to learn the same language;
• shared biopsychosocial conceptual framework; and
• basic understanding of pain mechanisms, conditions and principles of management.

Considering pain management as a whole, we can define numerous interfaces concerning competencies and tasks which may open up new perspectives on concepts of interprofessional education (Fragemann *et al.*, 2012). Pain experts should play a leading role in the care of patients suffering from acute, chronic or cancer pain based on interprofessional and monoprofessional core competencies. The definition of learning objectives considers the intersection

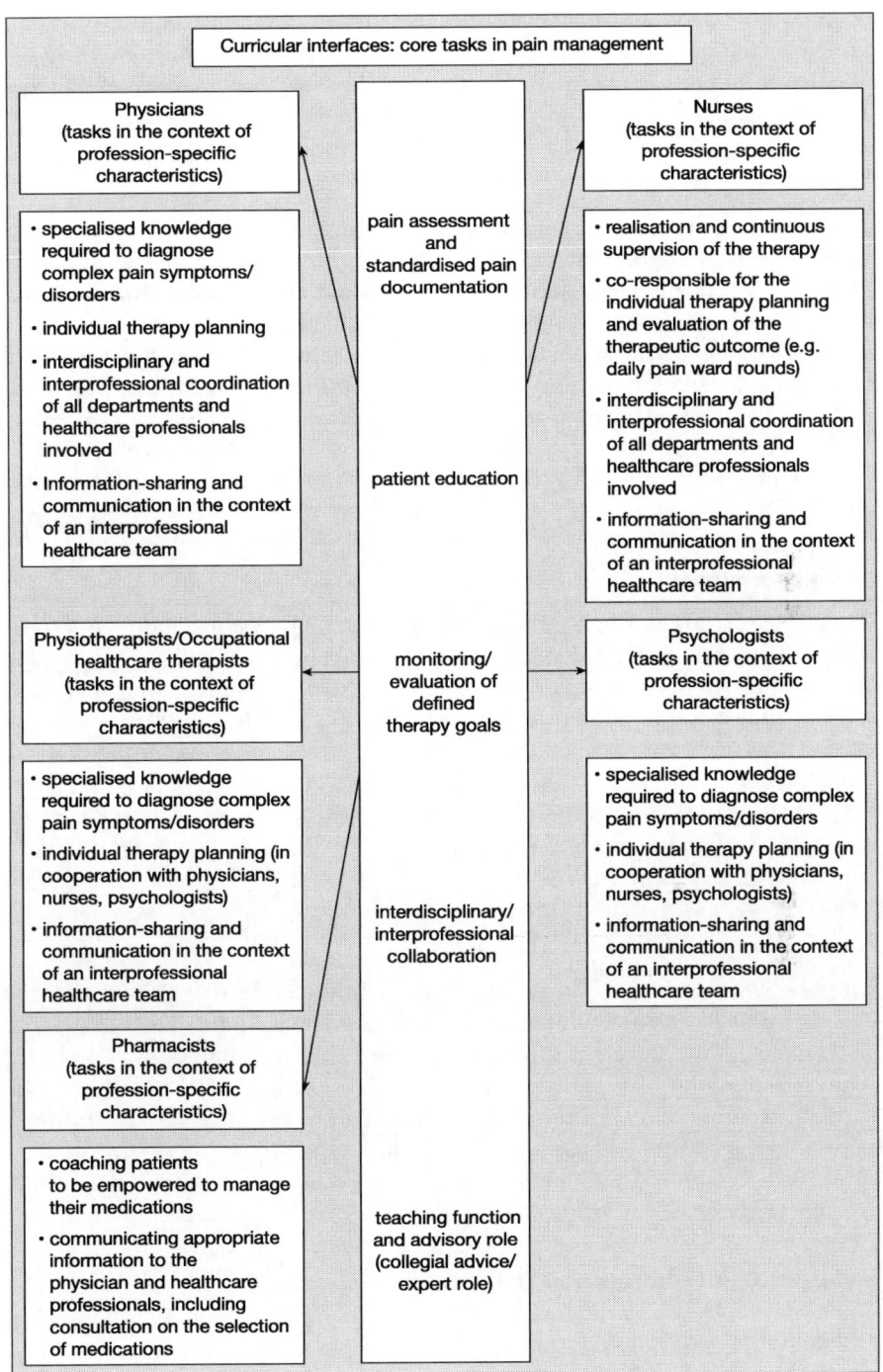

Figure 5.1 Curricular interfaces of healthcare professions in pain management

of tasks of all professions participating. This results in the definition of inter-professional core tasks that each healthcare professional must perform in practice. The tasks defined differ in the professionals' perspectives on patients and the degree of responsibility and detail (Fragemann *et al.*, 2012).

Teaching – course structure

The post-licensure pain curriculum is designed for clinically experienced healthcare professionals, such as physicians, nurses, psychologists, physio-therapists, occupational healthcare therapists and pharmacists. The 80-hour curriculum is scheduled across eight days with a maximum of ten hours per day in a single week. The 65-hour curriculum is divided into general fields of pain management for all types of professions and, additionally, into specialist fields of pain management for different healthcare professions to concretise topics according to their monoprofessional needs. The differentiation of the curriculum meets the formal requirements of the different professional associations.

Teaching strategies

Experience has shown that interprofessional teaching lessons require an inter-active element to foster a dialogue between different professional groups. The Regensburg Model provides presentations and interactive teaching methods, such as case studies, problem-centred discussions and the simulation of case conferences with real patients. The expert panel has established methodological guidelines to support teachers and to assure the quality of teaching. Regular team meetings, teachers' conferences and team brainstorming sessions create an atmosphere of transparency and networking for the members of the expert panel and other teachers participating.

Certification as a 'Pain Care Manager'

The post-licensure course is an 80-hour full-time course that provides parti-cipants with key qualifications in all areas of pain management. The course will be completed with a certificate declaring the title of 'Pain Care Manager', which is an interprofessional title. Upon completion of the sessions, all participants must take a written examination, shadow in a specialised institution with a heavy caseload of patients with pain, and complete a case report that summarises the principles of pain management from an interprofessional as well as from a monoprofessional point of view.

Evaluation of the course programme

Evaluation strategy

The purpose of the ongoing course evaluation is to assess the effectiveness of an interprofessional post-licensure programme in improving knowledge and

Integrative Core Curriculum
Interprofessional Pain Curriculum (post-licensure programme)

based on:
1) *Core Curriculum 'Special Pain Therapy' (post-licensure programme)*
   (German Chamber of Physicians)
2) *Integrated Pain Curriculum for Nurses (pre-licensure and post-licensure*
   nurse education programme) (German Pain Association)
3) *Core Curriculum for Professional Education in Pain (IASP Third Edition)*
4) *Curriculum on Pain for Schools of Occupational Therapy and*
   Physical Therapy

Modules [Interprofessional education (65 hrs)/monoprofessional education to meet the specific requirements of all types of professions (15 hrs)]

M1: Fields of activities in pain management: tasks and responsibilities
M2: Basic knowledge of pain management
M3: Diagnostic and therapeutic procedures
M4: Special pain therapy and pain disorders (acute and chronic pain symptoms)
M5: Interprofessional issues of pain management and related disciplines (psychiatry, psychology, language and cultural studies, nursing science and health sciences)
M6: Quality assurance concerning interprofessional pain management
M7: Legal aspects of pain management practices
M8: Practical module and simulation tool (the simulation module)
M9: Examination module (written final test; case report; opportunities for work shadowing)

Curriculum
- modules
- contents
- learning targets/ competencies
- teaching methods

Level 1

General fields of pain management for all types of professions (65 hrs)
M 1-8

Level 2

Interprofessional topics

integrated in the modules M1, M5-M8

- organising healthcare pathways for patients with acute or chronic pain
- establishing cooperative care structures
- considering roles, core competences and interfaces of related professions within the interdisciplinary team, special aspects and challenge of working in interdisciplinary teams
- considering interprofessional care standards and therapeutic algorithms
- reflecting interprofessional communication and collaboration related to process optimisation in the medical and patient care
- discussing ethical issues in pain management
- establishing and implementing control systems on good practice of pain management to ensure compliance with the evidence-based principles and guidelines (applied knowledge management)

Level 3

Specialist fields of pain management for different healthcare professions

(advanced training with the purpose of attaining additional qualifications e.g. 'Special Pain Therapy' (German Chamber of Physicians)

Figure 5.2 Overview of course structure and course contents

attitudes towards pain between professional groups which were academically trained and non-academically trained in their professional context. In the interest of promoting interprofessional education, the study also assessed experiences with interprofessional collaboration and learning. Based on a pre-post questionnaire design, effects were measured by (1) the German version of the 'Collaboration and Satisfaction About Care Decisions (CSACD)' developed by Baggs (1994) (permission for translation and validation was obtained; pre-test design), (2) the German version of The UWE (University of Western England) Entry-Level Interprofessional Questionnaire developed by Pollard (2004); the German version was translated by the Department of General Practice and Health Services Research, University of Heidelberg Hospital (pre–post-test design; Berger *et al.*, 2013) and (3) an adapted version of the 'Knowledge and Attitudes Survey Regarding Pain' developed by Ferrell and McCaffery (revised in 2004, and translated and validated by Gugler (2005); pre–post-test design).

Additionally, satisfaction with the programme, content and teaching methods was analysed with a course evaluation form (University Hospital Regensburg; post-test design). The study design aimed at collecting data from a total sample size of 250 students. The analyses were performed using IBM SPSS® software (IBM SPSS Statistics Standard). Data were analysed according to the total response. Paired student's t-tests were used for the 'UWE' and the adapted version of the 'Knowledge and Attitudes Survey Regarding Pain' to compare matched pre- and post-test scores, and unpaired t-tests were used to compare unmatched pre- and post-test scores. Descriptive analyses were completed for the 'UWE', CSACD and the course evaluation form. Summary statistics were calculated for the whole group and were calculated separately for particular groups of healthcare professions (Watt-Watson *et al.*, 2004). Qualitative descriptive analyses were generated by the categorization of data and were conducted for the open–ended questions of the course evaluation form and the individual conclusions of the case reports.

Interim results of the evaluation

A total of 49 healthcare professionals comprising 22 physicians, 25 nurses and 2 others completed the questionnaires (response rate 92 per cent). The sample was part of an ongoing study and represented interim results. The data collected were indicators to reveal a trend.

Attitudes, acceptance and potential effects of interprofessional education

The results are extractions of significant data from the *UWE Questionnaire* (not significant = p > 0.05). They demonstrate an agreement between all participants regarding the need for interprofessional education approaches to improve the quality of care (pre-/post-test > 90%). Both groups had an overall positive perception of interprofessional learning approaches (positive learning experience; p < 0.001). A significant majority of the participants were interested in attending interprofessional learning approaches again in the future (95%; p < 0.001).

Collaboration and satisfaction about care decisions (pre-test)

The CSACD (not significant = p > 0.05; 1 = strongly disagree; 7 = strongly agree) revealed that the interprofessional cooperation related to shared decision-making was experienced by approximately 50 per cent of the participants, as shown in Figure 5.3. Strong or very strong interprofessional cooperation and

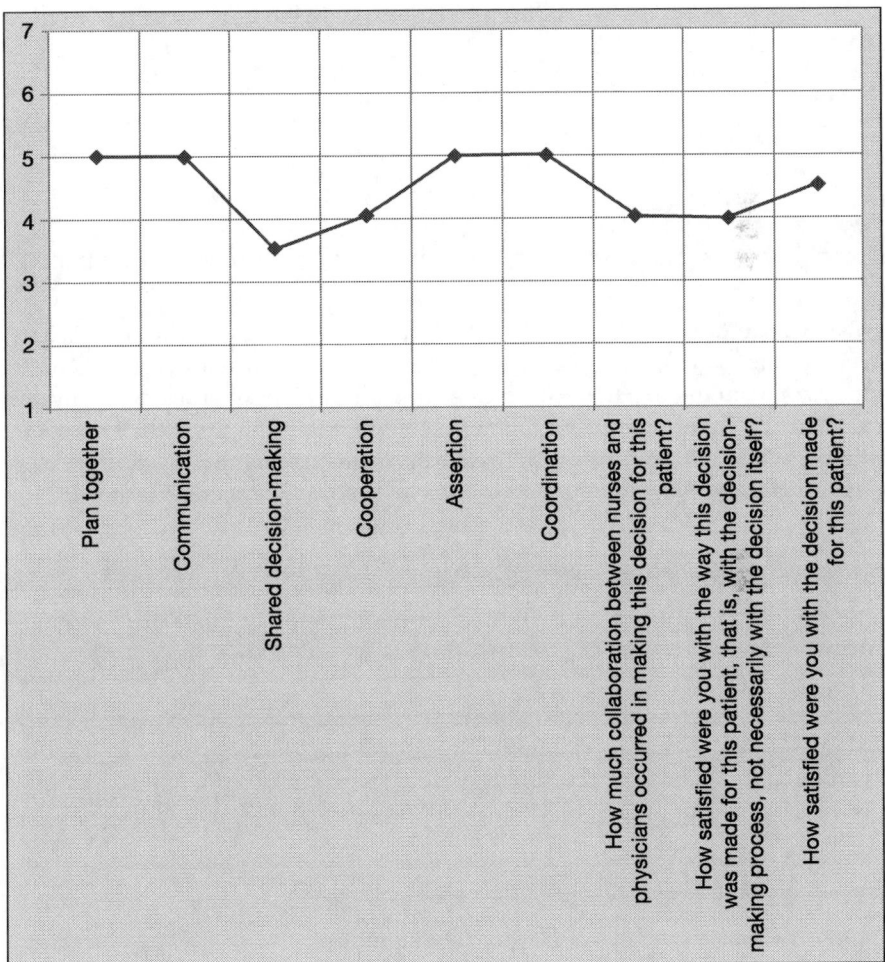

Figure 5.3 Collaboration and satisfaction about care decisions (CSACD)

Notes: Numbers are median values (pre-test)
Physicians vs. nurses: Chi^2 and t-test; t (df) = not significant (p > 0.05)

Table 5.1 Adapted version of the 'Knowledge and Attitudes Survey Regarding Pain'

Knowledge and attitudes toward pain and pain management

	N=47				t-test (p<0.05)
Pre-testing	Physicians (n=22)	Mean 38.90 (≈ 75%)	SD ±3.57		
	Nurses (n=25)	Mean 30.16 (≈ 58%)	SD ±5.94		
Post-testing	Physicians (n=22)	Mean 45.86 (≈ 88%)	SD ±3.04		p<0.001
	Nurses (n=25)	Mean 44.68 (≈ 87%)	SD ±3.52		p<0.001
Pre-testing vs. post-testing (Total)	Pre-testing	Mean 34.25 (≈ 65%)	Paired difference t-test Mean −10.97	SD± 6.53	p<0.001
	Post-testing	Mean 45.23 (≈ 87%)			

collaboration were experienced by less than 20 per cent of the participants. Overall, the participants evaluated the participative collaboration linked to aspects of planning together, communication and assertion with a median value of 5. There were no significant differences in the results between the two major groups (physicians and nurses). Shared decision-making was assessed with a median value of 3.5 and cooperation was assessed with a medium value of 4.

Knowledge and attitudes in pain management

The course evaluation was based on an adapted version of the 'Knowledge and Attitudes Survey Regarding Pain' (not significant = p > 0.05; Ferrell and McCaffery, 2004).

Physicians scored significantly better than nurses in the pre-test (p = 0.003; 75% vs. 61.5%), while in the post-test, both groups demonstrated a statistical approximation. The post-test scores of both were significantly higher than the pre-test knowledge scores (p < 0.001; 87% vs. 83%).

Participants' overall satisfaction with the course programme

The participants' overall satisfaction (not significant = p > 0.05; 1 = strongly agree; 5 = strongly disagree) in the course evaluation, as shown in Figure 5.4, demonstrated that there was significant agreement and a high degree of similarity between the two major groups of the course programme (physicians and nurses) related to learning effects and improved knowledge, teaching

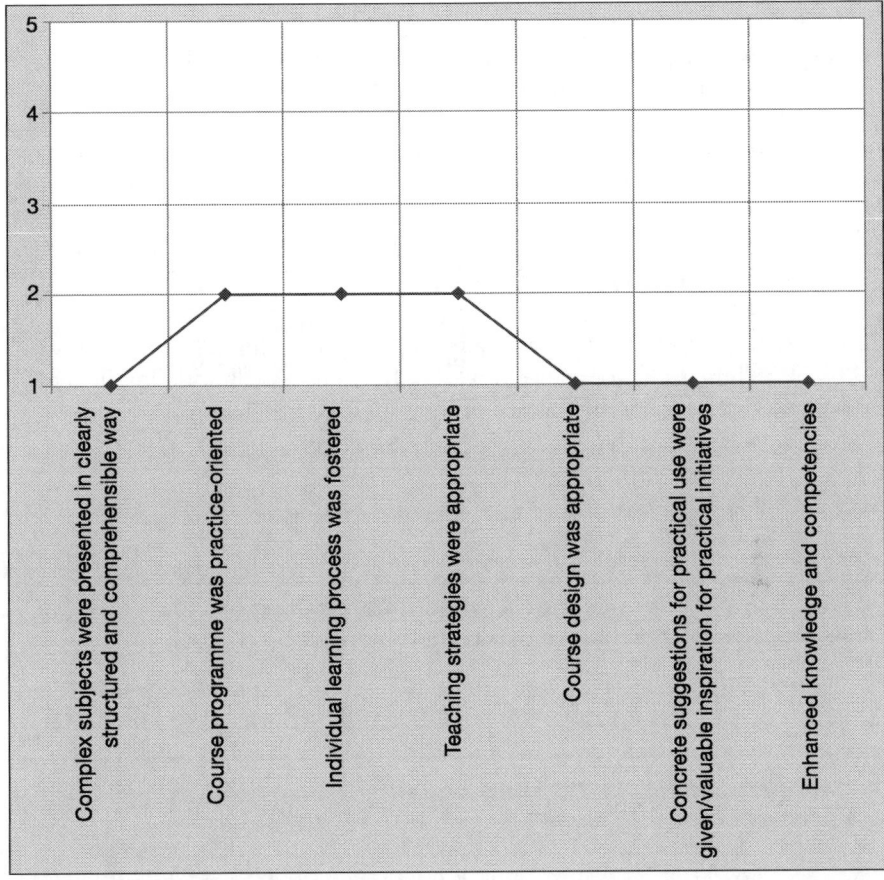

Figure 5.4 Participants' overall satisfaction as shown by course evaluation

Note: Numbers are median values

methods and the concept of interprofessional education itself. In general, the course programme was positively evaluated.

As shown in Boxes 5.1 and 5.2, the participants' comments provided understanding of how learning with other professionals was particularly helpful.

Discussion

The evaluation of the programme in accordance with other studies suggested a strong acceptance of interprofessional education approaches among healthcare professionals and encouraged the development of activities in the field of further education in German-speaking countries. All professional groups participating reported a significant improvement of knowledge and provided

---

Box 5.1 Summary response of final evaluations regarding the overall satisfaction with the course programme (open comments)

Mixed professions (summary responses)

- 'It is great to exchange expertise with other professions.' (Participant 9)
- 'I think it was useful to discuss and exercise aspects of pain management with other professions, as we have to collaborate in clinical practice.' (Participant 2)
- 'It was nice because I was networking with different professions, which helps to coordinate care and to exchange clinical experiences after completing the course programme.' (Participant 2)
- 'It was interesting to hear other professions' points of view and suggestions.' (Participant 3)

Box 5.2 Reflections of a physician (general practitioner) from a written case report

'Fortunately, two nurses from my practice environment did visit the same course programme. After completing the course programme, our communication was given at "the same" level. As an individual fighter, I experienced the multimodal and interprofessional therapy approach and proved myself step by step to be a creative team player.'

---

concrete suggestions for practical use. Valuable inspiration for practical initiatives was also elicited. The evaluation of all open feedback comments demonstrates the successful implementation of an interprofessional learning approach in the context of the course programme. The participants' perceptions of experiences focused on the chance to exchange expertise with other professions and the opportunity to network. Both aspects are key elements of interprofessional learning objectives and might foster the development of interprofessional competencies in the clinical context. In summary, the course programme was practice-oriented and an individual learning process was fostered. However, the results must be confirmed in a larger sample.

The study has some limitations. The two major groups that participated in the course programme were physicians and nurses. Consequently, the study cannot draw conclusions regarding other healthcare professions. The majority of the students attended the course programme as individuals, independently from their colleagues. Therefore, the evaluation cannot provide results regarding the transfer of interprofessional education objectives and competencies into practice. Furthermore, the evaluation did not assess the impact of inter-professional education on the quality of care (e.g. patient outcomes). There are a few external factors that might influence the quality of care in the context of interprofessional healthcare teams and make it difficult to prove the effects of interprofessional education.

Although various advantages of interprofessional education approaches have been cited in the literature, interprofessional education and collaboration present a few barriers related to the implementation of both interprofessional education and collaborative practice. In order to enhance the integration into practice, the University Hospital of Regensburg developed a project that aims at improving the quality of pain management and patient-centred care through interprofessional education and collaboration. Integrating research evidence into practice requires an educational strategy directed towards the inter-professional and interdisciplinary team as a whole, and there is probably a better chance of success if pain management representatives are defined within the team, clearly defining tasks and responsibilities (Fragemann and Wiese, 2014). Creating interprofessional algorithms for pain assessment and treatment may help to coordinate care and transfer concepts into clinical practice (Fragemann and Wiese, 2014).

In summary, interprofessional education is an appropriate concept to improve communication and collaboration between healthcare professionals of different training levels and enhances knowledge of pain management, but some of the implications of the recent findings in clinical practice still remain largely unclear (Dudley and Wiysonge, 2008). There has been some criticism of the fact that the quality of research on the topic is generally poor and the study designs are not comparable (Watt-Watson *et al.*, 2004, 2012; Reeves *et al.*, 2013). It is, therefore, essential to undertake further research on whether analysis should be performed based on standardised and comparable tools or by using appropriate qualitative research methods. Although the results of international empirical studies on the effects of interprofessional education differ, the findings, nevertheless, permit the conclusion that interprofessional learning groups will probably have a positive impact on the transformation from monoprofessional working habits to interprofessional team-building with effects on the quality of care (Carr and Watt-Watson, 2012; Watt-Watson *et al.*, 2012).

References

Aziz, Z., Chong Tek, L. and Yen Yen, P., 2011. The attitudes of medical, nursing and pharmacy students to IPE. *Social and Behavioral Sciences*, 29, pp. 639–45.

Baggs, J., 1994. Development of an instrument to measure collaboration and satisfaction about care decisions. *Journal of Advanced Nursing*, 20(1), pp. 176–82. (Permission for translation and validation for the questionnaire was obtained).

Berger, S., Hermann, K., Pollard, K., Stock, C., Szecsenyi, J. and Mahler, C., 2013. *Einstellungen von StudentInnen zu Kommunikation, Teamarbeit und interprofessionellem Lernen: Translation of the University of the West of England Interprofessional Questionnaire*

(UWE IP) into German. Abstract of 'Gesellschaft fuer Medizinische Ausbildung (GMA)'. Abstract of the annual conference of the GMA 2013. 26–28 September 2013. Graz, Austria. Düsseldorf: German Medical science GMS Publishing House; 2013. DocP06_07. Available through: <www.egms.de/static/resources/meetings/gma2013/Abstractband.pdf> [accessed 31 July 2015].

Bhamb, B., Brown, D., Hariharan, J., Anderson, J., Balousek, S. and Fleming, M.F., 2006. Survey of select practice behaviours by primary care physicians on the use of opioids for chronic pain. *Current Medical Research Opinion*, 22(9), pp. 1859–65.

Bredanger, S., Hege-Scheuing, G., Karst, M., Kopf, A., Michel, S., Ruschulte, H.B. *et al.*, 2008. *Kerncurriculum Schmerztherapie für die Lehre für das Querschnittfach Schmerztherapie nach der neuen AO. Erarbeitet durch die Ad-hoc-Kommission 'Studienordnungen'.* Available through: <www.dgss.org/fileadmin/pdf/6_KerncurriculumDeutsch_2009_07_16_Kurzversion_final_ohneDEGAM.pdf> [accessed 20 April 2015].

Breivik, H., Collett, B., Ventafridda, V., Cohen, R. and Gallacher, D., 2006. Survey of chronic pain in Europe: prevalence, impact on daily life, and treatment. *European Journal of Pain*, 10(4), pp. 287–333.

Briggs, E.V., 2014. Pain care: overhaul education for the next generation. *Nursing Times*, [online] 17 January. Available through: <www.nursingtimes.net> [accessed 24 February 2015].

Briggs, E.V., Carr, E.C. and Whittaker, M.S., 2011. Survey of undergraduate pain curricula for healthcare professionals in the United Kingdom. *European Journal of Pain*, 15, pp. 789–95.

Burke, S. and Shorten, G.D., 2009. When pain after surgery doesn't go away. . . . *Biochemical Society Transactions*, 37, pp. 318–22.

CAIPE: Centre for the Advancement of Interprofessional Education, 2002. Defining interprofessional education. Available through: <www.caipe.org.uk/about-us/defining-ipe> [accessed 24 February 2015].

Carpenter, J., 1995. Doctors and nurses. Stereotypes and stereotype change in IPE. *Journal of Interprofessional Care*, 9(2), pp. 151–61.

Carr, E.C.J., 2003. Improving pain management through interprofessional education: evaluation of a pilot project. *Learning in Health and Social Care*, 2(1), pp. 6–17.

Carr, E.C.J. and Watt-Watson, J. 2012. Interprofessional pain education: definitions, exemplars and future directions. *British Journal of Pain*, 6(2), pp. 59–65.

D'Amour, D., 2005. The conceptual basis for interprofessional collaboration: core concepts and theoretical frameworks. *Journal of Interprofessional Care*, 19(1), pp. 116–31.

D'Amour, D. and Oandasan, I., 2005. Interprofessionality as the field of inter-professional practice and IPE: an emerging concept. *Journal of Interprofessional Care*, 1, pp. 8–20.

Deandrea, S., 2008. Prevalence of undertreatment in cancer pain. A review of published literature. *Annals of Oncology*, 19, pp. 1985–91.

Dudley, L. and Wiysonge, C.S., 2008. Does interprofessional education improve professional practice and health care outcomes? A SUPPORT summary of a systematic review. Available through: <http://supportsummaries.org/support-summaries/show/does-interprofessional-education-improve-professional-practice-and-health-care-outcomesa> [accessed 14 July 2015].

Ferrell, B.F. and McCaffery, M., 2004. Knowledge and Attitudes Survey Regarding Pain developed by B.F. Ferrell and M. McCaffery. Revised 2004, translated and validated by Gugler, E., 2005. Available through: <http://prc.coh.org> [accessed 10 February 2013].

Fragemann, K. and Wiese, C.H.R., 2011. Weiterbildung in der Schmerztherapie – Stand mono- und interprofessioneller Konzepte im deutschsprachigen Raum. Abstract of *German Pain Congress 2011.* Mannheim, Germany, 5–8 October 2011. *Schmerz*, 1, pp. 1–164.

Fragemann, K. and Wiese, C., 2014. Pain education policies and initiatives in Europe. *Journal of Pain & Palliative Care Pharmacotherapy*, 28(4), pp. 402–3.

Fragemann, K., Meyer, N., Graf, B.M. and Wiese, C.H., 2012. Interprofessional education in pain management. Development strategies for an interprofessional core curriculum for health professionals in German-speaking countries. *Schmerz*, 26, pp. 369–82.

German Pain Association (Deutsche Schmerzgesellschaft e.V.), 2012. Medizinische Fakultaten in denen das Deutsche Schmerzgesellschaft e.V. Curriculum implementiert ist. Available through: <www.dgss.org/aus-weiter-fortbildung/curriculare-lehre/> [accessed 19 February 2015].

Gilbert, H.V., Yan, J. and Hoffman, S.J., 2010. A WHO report: framework for action on interprofessional education and collaborative practice. *Journal of Allied Health*, 39(1), pp. 196–7.

Gugler, E., 2005. *Wissen und Einstellung diplomierter Pflegefachpersonen zum Schmerzmanagement.* Master's thesis. WE'G Aarau, Switzerland, and Maastricht University, the Netherlands.

Hammick, M., Freeth, D., Koppel, I., Reeves, S. and Barr, H., 2007. A best evidence systematic review of IPE: BEME Guide no. 9. *Medical Teacher*, 29, pp. 735–51.

Hertweck, M.L., Hawkins, S.R., Bednarek, M.L., Goreczny, A.J., Schreiber, J.L. and Sterrett, S.E., 2012. Attitudes toward interprofessional education among health care professions graduate students. *Journal of Physician Assistant Education*, 23, pp. 8–15.

Hunter, J., Watt-Watson, J., McGillion, M., Raman-Wilms, L., Cockburn, L., Lax, L. *et al.*, 2008. An interfaculty pain curriculum: lessons learned from six years experience. *Pain*, 140, pp. 74–86.

IASP: International Association of the Study of Pain, 2012. Interprofessional Pain Curriculum Outline, 2012. Available through: <www.iasp-pain.org/Education/CurriculumDetail.aspx?ItemNumber=2057> [accessed 12 February 2014].

IASP: International Association for the Study of Pain, 2015. Curricula. Available through: <www.iasp-pain.org/Education/CurriculaList.aspx?navItemNumber=647> [accessed 26 August 2015].

Irajpour, A., 2006. Interprofessional education: a facilitator to enhance pain management? *Journal of Interprofessional Care*, 20(6), pp. 675–8.

Johnson, M., Collett, B. and Castro-Lopes, J.M., 2013. The challenges of pain management in primary care: a pan-European survey. *Journal of Pain Research*, 6, pp. 393–401.

Kern, D.E., Thomas, P.A., Howard, D.M. and Bass, E.B., 1998. *Curriculum development for medical education: a six-step approach.* Baltimore, MD: Johns Hopkins University Press.

Lin, P.C., Chiang, H.W., Chiang, T.T. and Chen, C.S., 2008. Pain management: evaluating the effectiveness of an educational programme for surgical nursing staff. *Journal of Clinical Nursing*, 1(15), pp. 2022–31.

Maier, C., Nestler, N., Richter, H., Hardinghaus, W., Pogatzki-Zahn, E., Zenz, M. and Osterbrink, J., 2010. The quality of pain management in German hospitals. *Deutsches Ärzteblatt International*, 107, pp. 607–14.

McFadyen, A.K., Webster, V., Strachan, K., Figgins, E., Brown, H. and McKechnie, J., 2005. The readiness for IPE scale: a possible more stable subscale model for the original version of RIPLS. *Journal of Interprofessional Care*, 19, pp. 595–603.

Mundipharma, 2013. A blueprint for pain education – the APPEAL study. Mundipharma data file. Available through: <www.mundipharma.com/docs/default-source/default-document-library/appeal-study-backgrounder-%28final-03-10-13%29.pdf?sfvrsn=0> [accessed 26 August 2015].

Pargeon, K.L. and Hailey, B.J., 1999. Barriers to effective pain management: a review of the literature. *Journal of Pain Symptom Management*, 18, pp. 358–68.

Pflughaupt, M., Scharnagel, R., Gossrau, G., Kaiser, U., Koch, T. and Sabatowski, R., 2010. Befragung schmerztherapeutisch interessierter Ärzte zum Umgang mit Opioiden. *Schmerz*, 24(3), pp. 267–75.

Pollard, K., 2004. The UWE (University of Western England) Entry-Level Interprofessional Questionnaire, developed by K. Pollard, 2004. German version translated by Dept. of General Practice and Health Services Research, University of Heidelberg Hospital. Original Version. Data on file.

Pollard, K. and Miers, M., 2008. From students to professionals: results of a longitudinal study of attitudes to pre-qualifying collaborative learning and working in health and social care in the United Kingdom. *Journal of Interprofessional Care*, 22(4), pp. 399–416.

Pollard, K., Sellman, D. and Thomas, J., 2014. The need for interprofessional working. In: J. Thomas, K. Pollard, D. Sellman, eds., *Interprofessional working in health and social care: professional perspectives*. Second edition. Basingstoke: Palgrave Macmillan, pp. 9–21.

Reeves, S., Perrier, L., Goldman, J., Freeth, D. and Zwarenstein, M., 2013. Interprofessional education: effects on professional practice and healthcare outcomes (update). *Cochrane Database of Systematic Reviews*, March, 28(3), p. CD002213. doi: 10.1002/14651858.CD002213.pub3.

Strickland, J.M., Huskey, A. and Brushwood, D.B., 2007. Pharmacist–physician collaboration in pain management practice. *Journal of Opioid Management*, 3(6), pp. 295–301.

The Medical Association of North Rhine [ÄkNo], 2014. Medizinische Fakultaeten und Fachschaften in Deutschland, Oesterreich und der Schweiz. Available through: <www.aekno.de/page.asp?pageID=5297> [accessed 24 February 2014].

van den Beuken-van Everdingen, M.H., de Rijke, J.M., Kessels, A.G., Schouten, H.C., van Kleef, M. and Patijn, J., 2007. Prevalence of pain in patients with cancer: a systematic review of the past 40 years. *Annals of Oncology*, 18, pp. 1437–49.

Watt-Watson, J., Hunter, J., Pennefather, P., Librach, L., Raman-Wilms, L., Schreiber, M. *et al.*, 2004. An integrated undergraduate pain curriculum, based on IASP curricula, for six health science faculties. *Pain*, 110, pp. 140–8.

Watt-Watson, J., Siddall, P.J. and Carr, E., 2012. Interprofessional pain education: the road to successful pain management outcomes. *Pain Management*, 2(5), pp. 417–20.

WHO: World Health Organization, 1988. *Learning together to work together for health. Report of a WHO study group on multiprofessional education for health personnel.* The Team Approach Technical Report Series 769. [pdf] Geneva, Switzerland. Available through: <http://whqlibdoc.who.int/trs/WHO_TRS_769.pdf> [accessed 20 April 2015].

Zwarenstein, M., Reeves, S. and Perrier, L., 2005. Effectiveness of pre-licensure interprofessional education and post-licensure collaborative interventions. *Journal of Interprofessional Care*, 19(1), pp. 148–65.

Zwarenstein, M., Goldman, J. and Reeves, S., 2009. Interprofessional collaboration: effects of practice-based interventions on professional practice and healthcare outcomes. *Cochrane Database Systematic Reviews*, July 8(3), p. CD000072.

Part III

Transformation of healthcare professions

6 Professionalism of the health workforce in Ukraine

Tetiana Stepurko, Alona Goroshko and Paolo Carlo Belli

Introduction

Professionalism is closely related to access and quality of care (Passi *et al.*, 2010). The concept of professionalism in the medical field is constructed from a variety of characteristics, for example, excellence, respect of others, altruism, duty, accountability, and honour or integrity (Chisholm *et al.*, 2006), as well as clinical competence (Veloski *et al.*, 2005). Recent trends have been moving from the individual to the institutional dimensions: professionalism should be inculcated within medical schools with complete integration of a culture of professionalism' (Passi *et al.*, 2010, p. 20). Indeed, a deeper look into the culture and context contributes to the interpretation of 'professionalism' in a society as 'certain elements that characterize the nature of medical practice are key to providing a contextual understanding of medical professionalism', underlined by Swick (2000, p. 613). In particular, institutions, social expectations and the nature of their transition frame the behaviour and responsibility of healthcare service providers within any one country or context.

Professionalism as an important characteristic of healthcare providers is often expected and valued by consumers. Lack of professionalism, for example, is recognised as the fourth most problematic area of the Romanian health-care system, while corruption, lack of interest of medical staff and lack of modern medical equipment are the top three on the list (Fărcăşanu, 2010). These challenges of the system of healthcare service provision are relevant for most countries in the Eastern European region, however, their degree differs (Rechel and McKee, 2009; Pavlova *et al.*, 2012).

A rise in 'self-help' coping strategies has been noticed in Ukraine during sociopolitical changes (Williams and Onoschenko, 2013; Polese, 2014) as a response to the distrust and scepticism toward public institutions and to insufficient funding with inadequate allocative efficiency (Polese and Stepurko, 2016). Moreover, Ukraine shows high rates of corruption, low rates of political stability and a very moderate level of economic development and health expenditure.[1] The burden of healthcare service financing has shifted to patients and their families: about 18 per cent have to borrow money or sell assets and about 60 per cent of Ukrainian respondents report on forgoing healthcare services (Tambor *et al.*, 2014). However, despite having widespread quasi-formal and informal patient payments, high private expenditure is not recognised as problematic by key stakeholders in Ukraine (Gryga *et al.*, 2010; Stepurko *et al.*, 2013). By and large, a mixture of practices conducted under 'multiple moralities' (Wanner, 2005, p. 530) and the extensive use of networks (Ledeneva, 1998) are intertwined in the healthcare system and other public services provision.

Furthermore, health outcomes in Ukraine remain poor: life expectancy at birth increased by only one year between 1970 and 2010, and is currently 71 years (66 for men and 76 for women), which is approximately six years lower than the WHO European region average (WHO, 2013). Ukraine has not shown significant progress in the strengthening of primary healthcare (General Practitioner practices), the reduction of hospital capacity (9.0 hospital beds per 1,000 population in Ukraine in contrast to 6.5 in Poland, 6.2 in Moldova and 6.1 in Romania; WHO, 2013), the improvement of quality and equity in healthcare provision, or improvements in cost–effectiveness. Primary healthcare delivery has remained essentially the way it was, with a large network of underperforming urban and rural polyclinics, women's consultation clinics, poorly equipped rural physicians' ambulatories, polyclinic units in urban hospitals and outpatient departments in rural hospitals. In fact, primary care physicians are consulted only for minor complaints, and patients have obtained care from a specialist without any formal referral for decades. The lack of an effective referral system and the absence of clear 'care pathways' and post-discharge care protocols contribute to costly (and avoidable) admissions and readmissions for mostly non–communicable diseases.

In contrast to other countries in Eastern Europe, Ukraine has not switched from the system of central planning and declared free–of–charge healthcare to a decentralised system with a health insurance fund (Danyliv *et al.*, 2012; Lekhan *et al.*, 2015). This suggests that the Ukrainian healthcare system has a low potential for change and effective decision-making. Moreover, the country has experienced numerous appointments of Ministers of Health during the last decade (about ten appointments with an average length of stay of 1–1.5 years), which partly explains the uneven character of healthcare sector development.

Taking into account the specific context of the Ukrainian healthcare system, we question how professionalism within it is constructed. We particularly aim to identify both good and challenging practices as well as administrative approaches for assuring healthcare professionalism at Ukrainian public facilities.

Methodology

In this chapter, we study the topic of professionalism of the Ukrainian health workforce and aspects of the environment that ensure the enhancement of professionalism, using an ethnographic approach and qualitative data collected through the 'Governance in healthcare in Ukraine' research project (Belli, Dzygyr and Maynzyuk, 2015). This study was initiated by the World Bank and implemented in cooperation with analytical and sociological organisations. The wider frame of the study aimed to compare the legislative framework with *de facto* practices that exist in healthcare facilities and healthcare governance at the local level. The explorative–descriptive research approach allows us to include a special look in this chapter at medical professionalism and the obstacles related to its enhancement.

Empirical data for this project was collected through structured interviews conducted with several groups of respondents:

- healthcare providers (82 respondents): medical doctors, nurses, chief nurses;
- administrators of healthcare facilities (25 respondents): heads of facility departments and chief doctors, as well as deputies of chief doctors;
- regional policy-makers (11 respondents): *oblast* and *rayon* (both are administrative areas of Ukraine) heads or representatives of healthcare departments.

The scope of the empirical study covered five regions of Ukraine, with Central Ukraine represented by Kyiv, the capital (where the research instrument was pretested), Vinnitsa and Poltava regions, Western Ukraine represented by Lviv region and Eastern Ukraine represented by Luhansk region. The regions were selected for the study based on (a) the availability of reliable contact points (to assure data quality and reliability in terms of potentially sensitive topic) and also (b) representation of regions of different cultural and geographical areas of Ukraine and of regional peculiarities of healthcare system provision (for example, status of pilot *oblast* in healthcare reform launched in 2010). Snowball and convenience sampling methods were applied for each region, its facilities and medical staff, as well as the administrative body's selection of representatives. The most important condition for recruiting the respondent was more than two-years' working experience in the position.

The research instrument was developed by the team of the researchers and included three major sections on: (a) human resources, (b) planning, budgeting and financing, and (c) medical information. A mixture of open- and closed-ended questions were presented in the questionnaire, since both stories about personal work experience and quantitative estimations of the spread of practices were important. The instrument was pretested with an empirical data collection in the summer and autumn of 2012. Face-to-face interviews based on the questionnaire developed with specific parts for each group of respondents were considered the most appropriate data collection mode, as they allowed for the study of respondents' individual unique experiences and attitudes, as well as aspects of the quality of governance perceived and its procedures. Furthermore, questions on non-transparent and corruptible (or bribing) practices were included in the research agenda as additional means to ensure data validity under the topic sensitivity. As is shown in Box 6.1, we paid special attention to sensitive questions of the questionnaire by asking questions on both personal

---

Box 6.1   Example of the sensitive questions asked in the study

(*Type A question*) Please describe the usual practices followed in the hiring of medical staff, according to your experience – doctors, nurses (are there any differences?)

(*Type B question*) In your experience, which of the following criteria are more important when medical doctors/nurses/other staff are appointed? Show card. Ask respondent to rank answers (1 – most important), add answers to the table.

- Knowledge, skills and capacity
- Performance in previous relevant employment
- Education
- Years of experience
- Loyalty to hospital management (no criticism)
- Political affiliations
- Connections (factors of interpersonal nature – being friends, old colleagues; family ties; being recommended by such people)
- Other. Specify: _____

(*Type C question*) There is a wide-spread public belief nowadays that it's impossible for a doctor to get a job without using some private connections to an employer or authorities, or paying money. Do you know of any case that contradicts this view (among your colleagues or doctors you know)?

(*Type D question*) What would you estimate to be the share of people whom you know who get a job mostly because of their merits (knowledge, experience and other professional qualities) and not because of any other factors?

---

experience and perceived experience of others, as well as questions of similar content but of different connotations and changed wording (Tourangeau and Smith, 1996).

Face-to-face interviews were mostly conducted at the facility where the respondent worked, though a minority of respondents agreed to meet for an interview in a public place. The duration of an interview with medical personnel was about one hour and about two hours with administrators. Each interview was audio recorded with the respondent's approval. A small cash compensation was provided for virtually all medical staff and facility administrators who were respondents to provide the motivation to accept the survey invitation. Payment was given at the end of the conversation. A direct cash payment as stimulus to public servants, for example, representatives of health departments, was not used due to national anti–corruption policies. Confidentiality was guaranteed to all respondents. The individuals participated in the study on a voluntary basis. Two researchers (co–authors of the paper) analysed the data qualitatively and independently from each other without using computer software as a triangulation at the stage of qualitative data interpretation.

Results

The results of the study suggest the presence of problematic aspects of the environment from which healthcare professionalism originates. Here, we describe practices and perceptions reported by healthcare providers and administrators in several fields related to professionalism: the improvement of clinical and service qualification of providers, appointments and the job appraisal system.

Postgraduate medical education

Specialised state medical courses are basic obligatory and regular (every five years) education for physicians during their career. These courses are essential for promotion to higher medical categories. The certificate regarding state postgraduate education is issued to medical doctors who pass computer–assisted tests and who collect enough points during a certain period of time (a so-called 'cumulative point system'). In our study, physicians underlined the challenges related to the transparency of state attestation that has been partially overcome by the introduction of computer–assisted exams, which minimise the personal influence of the examiner. Most of the respondents consider the state courses a formality with minor impact on real knowledge and skills, although the courses are seen as a possibility to extend one's professional network via communication with colleagues from other regions. The participation in these courses is not very valued by facility administration (chief doctors' comments) since the curricula of the courses are rather theoretical and not relevant to the practice.

We notice positive experience of medical doctors (respondents) concerning educational events which are organised in healthcare facilities. Such seminars, lectures and workshops are mostly initiated by the administration of the facility – by the chief nurse, the head of department or the chief doctor. It is important to note that these training sessions are usually implemented with the support of other institutions, for example, international organisations, projects and pharmaceutical companies. In–facility short–term and irregular training sessions are considered by physicians as a more effective way of getting relevant knowledge compared to the previous form of professional postgraduate education. Although the share of answers is virtually the same between the two types of training, the comments about internal training are more positive and less formal. However, some physicians dispute the high quality of both of these training sessions and state courses and argue that the design of educational activities does not always tackle the need for updated knowledge and skills for narrow specialities:

> Those who graduated 20 years ago can be happy with this kind of course as well as with each conference. But for those who graduated two years ago and who constantly read medical literature, these events are not so attractive because of the lack of new information – I constantly hear repetitive information here.
>
> (Lugansk city, physician, in-patient facility)

In terms of improving the skills and knowledge of medical personnel, 'external' education – that is, outside the state system of postgraduate education and in-facility events – is more positively perceived by the majority of the respondents. Indeed, such 'master-classes' and conferences are perceived as real professional development. However, these workshops and conferences which they perceive as worth attending are paid for by medical doctors personally out of their own pockets. Other sources to fund participation in external events come from the pharmaceutical industry. In rare cases, the expenses are shared with a public healthcare facility (for example, the participation fee is paid by the employee, while travel costs and *per diems* are covered by the facility).

Some physicians also report hiding their participation in additional educational activities from the administration: they ask for days off work or holidays without mentioning the real purpose. Although the motives for avoiding mentioning education as a purpose of leave are rarely discussed, several answers provide clear indications of the unwillingness of facility administration to manage gaps in service provision when the doctors are engaged in activities outside the facility. Meanwhile, physicians participating in this study find 'private' (non-government) external training as the only possibility to get the relevant, modern and essential knowledge to update their professional skills. A few physicians admit that the best effect on professional growth is participation in international educational events (outside of the country), but this option is a rather expensive one and the use of the English language at these events creates a barrier. However, such valuable activities for medical practice often have very little impact on the formal side of promotion: 'private' training does not carry any points for state attestation and, therefore, does not contribute to achieving higher categorisation and, consequently, has little impact on the formal salary of a physician.

Thus, the process of the professional development of physicians is constructed mostly at the initiative of the doctor, who invests substantial personal financial capital (which is, however, often earned via informal patient payments), and is rarely initiated by the administration of the healthcare facility.

Job appointments at healthcare facilities

Access to information concerning vacancies can be characterised as a 'trade secret', as such information is quite often seen as a resource of the administration. Indeed, a large share of health workers suggest that a major bottle-neck in the field of employment is the lack of open and accessible information on available vacancies:

> In our facility we do not have vacant job positions, but from time to time new staff appears [. . .] nobody informs others how they have got that position but I am sure they are employed with a reason behind it [. . .] My son had to move to Zhytomyr because we could not find any vacant position in Lviv as here the competition among physicians is extremely high.
>
> (Lviv city, physician, in-patient facility)

Furthermore, instead of creating a good platform for engaging the best staff at the facility and, therefore, stimulating a competitive atmosphere at the point of entry, chief doctors or other representatives of the administration of some healthcare facilities are actively involved in maintaining the old-style system of appointments. The study shows that job positions are mostly 'offered' by the chief doctor to some preselected medical doctors in cities. There is no formal procedure to register and appraise the candidate's application, and selection is mostly done by the chief doctor and head of department without any standard criteria:

> To be honest, there are two pathways for appointment: an official way – a nice one, and an unofficial one that works in 50% of cases. A medical student after graduation is practically nobody and nobody wants to take him into a vacant position. Such students can just work in the emergency room of the facility or as an outpatient service provider in a rural area. It is the only possible job position for those who do not use 'gratitude' [. . .] But everything else is achieved because of 'gratitude' or friendship. If a person has a higher professional level, he has more options for appointment [. . .] Still, here we have a person at the facility with a minor knowledge about prescriptions and treatment, as well as about medical information keeping, but somehow she has a fairly high position. Although, when we ask her a question, she cannot adequately respond and always sends us to get consultation from other colleagues.
>
> (Kyiv city, physician, outpatient facility)

Indeed, recently graduated medical doctors and nurses point to *napravlennia* (referral) to a facility as a means of securing a job after graduation. Such referrals are taken at the *oblast* or *rayon* health department. We identified several respondents who shared their experiences about the formal procedure of referral, which can also be supplemented by informal practices in order to avoid referral to rural area. Those who work in *rayon* hospitals indicate that they are able to get a referral without either problems or informal agreements, in contrast to healthcare staff, who have a more prestigious place of work, for example, in cities or at in-patient departments.

Among physicians and nurses, those who work in cities have wider limits in the healthcare human resource market, as they show better familiarity with opportunities for changing job positions than do physicians from *rayon* facilities. The latter perceive the question about the experience of applying for a job position only within the context of '*rozpodil*' ('assignment' – obligatory referral to a certain healthcare facility as directed by the state):

> I have no idea about hiring procedures. I got this job about 30 years ago when I graduated from the university and I received a referral. I think the same procedure is applied now. Young physicians who work at our facility say they have come here due to referral.
>
> (Vinnitsa region, physician, in-patient facility)

The respondents consider knowledge, skills (according to 22 out of 41 physicians and 3 out of 16 nurses) and education (according to 12 out of 41 physicians and 7 out of 16 nurses) as the most important criteria for appointment, while personal connections are the main source for information about vacant positions (according to 38 out of 71 respondents from the physician–nurse subgroup). Such inconsistency in the respondents' answers can be explained by chief doctors' and department heads' interest in hiring staff with good knowledge and skills because it will lead to higher performance indicators for the department as well as the satisfaction of patients and low complaint rates. However, candidates for vacant positions are often chosen from the personal network of the administration in line with the need to have loyal employees. It may not exclude an informal payment to a chief doctor for the opportunity to be hired:

> The chief doctor selects really qualified staff, but such conditions are created for having applicants from a narrow circle, so a stranger cannot appear in the list for interview with the chief. Or it should be a kind of benefit to the administration. Qualities are important, but there should still be some connection. The chief doctor will take only the best of those whom he knows, it is not a thoughtless decision.
>
> (Vinnitsa city, physician, in-patient facility)

Overall, these major problems in attaining a position – lack of information and lack of transparent criteria – are noticed by physicians and nurses. The opinions of employees are quite different when they are asked to estimate the ease of searching and getting an appropriate position: some report quite easy pathways to reach the final appointment, while others note that they needed several years to get the position they have now. Possibly, the specialisation of the physician contributes to the huge variation in the answers: several of the respondents who are dentists, for example, do not recall problematic issues, since the private sector is quite developed in that field, while cardiologists and endocrinologists have a long path to travel to reach their desired position.

All groups of respondents agree that there is a much easier path for job appointment for nurses compared to physicians, due to nurses' lower responsibility and lower access to informal income sources. These and other factors, for example, working conditions, make the position and profession unattractive.

However, there is variation in the formal regulations in the regions. In Vinnitsa city, for example, relatively recent regulations for the hiring of physicians have been introduced: transparency of medical doctors' appointments has been considered as the goal of this intervention. In particular, information about the vacancy is published in the newspaper and on a web page, the list of documents for the job application are collected at the city health department, and then, a committee of professors and chief doctors (about 15 committee members) interviews each applicant. Chief doctors and administration representatives find this 'open competition' to be a fair and transparent procedure; however, virtually all physicians who work in Vinnitsa's city healthcare facilities and interviewed for this study mention 'open competition' with great scepticism, since the procedure has inherited earlier practices which include bribery and/or social connections.

> A web-page of the *miskarda* [city council] offers application forms, and then we wait for the competition. We present a CV, diploma, its supplement, the certificate of internship. I personally paid the chief doctor, but personal connections and communicable skills are also important. Social connections play an essential role in our city – without such connections it is impossible to live. All arrangements involve personal connections and agreements. I have a family where all members are physicians and we do not know anyone who applied for a job without a personal connection, but in the Soviet Union it was not so deep-rooted.
>
> (Vinnitsa city, physician, in-patient facility)

In short, the overall system of job appointments remains uncertain, with an absence of clear and transparent rules and procedures, and there is a prevalent use of informal practices. Professionalism in each specific case of appointment may have a different level of importance, depending on the type of position and the administrator's human resource typical practices.

Job appraisal system

The lack of a systematic approach in professionalism enhancement is also noticeable in performance appraisal procedures at the facility level. Generally, the majority of chief doctors interviewed in our study were able to describe key principles of the appraisal system at their organisation in detail. In most cases, the appraisal system in health facilities represented the combination of formal and informal approaches. In some of the departments, the performance indicators are chosen and collected, and summarised at the facility level. The representatives of the facility administration, as well as doctors and nurses, assume that these scores are used to stimulate the performance of the department. In particular, one chief doctor of a city in-patient facility mentioned that when he gets an offer to host any kind of equipment, those who perform better have a greater probability of getting it, though such situations occur rarely. The formal appraisal methods are mandatory for all facilities in the country, whereas informal appraisal procedures can be established in a variety of ways, including single penalty measures with no rewards for good performance.

> Appraisal, it is a rare practice. If you work well, everybody just keeps silent. But if you start making mistakes [*kosyachyt*], then the punishments will surely reach you and it varies from 'come to my office' to losing a bonus for the month and even for the year. There are doctors who – for whatever reasons – have been prohibited from signing sick leaves. So they treat patients, and then they show them to another physician who has the right to issue the sick leave.
>
> (Kyiv city, physician, outpatient facility)

The following tools are mentioned particularly concerning the informal part of job appraisal: informal conversations with the department head or with the chief doctor; night shifts as a sanction; prohibition to issue sick leave, and so on. Overall, the performance assessment is mostly associated with punishment rather than with rewarding for good performance. In other words, 'a carrot and stick' motivation principle is used, but the carrot is too small to be attractive, while the stick is often used. Moreover, informal methods to punish personnel are also reflected in formal calculations of bonuses (overall salary) and less often in possibilities to participate in training (as has been mentioned above, the administration is rarely informed by physicians about their additional education).

It is interesting, however, that facility administration is very limited in available ('fully legal') tools to stimulate or to sanction the performance of their employees and, therefore, we observed a huge variation in human resource decisions. In particular, we identified a case of the use of state attestation as a sanction tool for the physician in response to a patient complaint.

> One physician had a conflict with the patient. We assumed that the doctor violated ethics and did not show relevant qualifications, so we sent him for recertification in the area. And if his category is not confirmed, he will lose a part of his wage. They [the state attestation committee] understand that if we send someone for recertification without a good recommendation then there are reasons. We cannot reduce his salary directly [. . .]. Rewards are not seen as a tool to influence salary as we cannot cancel premiums for continuity of employment. We may forbid a person from having two

positions at the facility [. . .] the only way to influence the situation – to challenge a category if he made a mistake in professional work, and if you do not like something that is not comfortable for you – it is impossible to do anything.

(Poltava region, head of department, outpatient facility)

However, personnel mistakes are rarely revealed publicly and are usually discussed at facility meetings. The principle of *krugova poruka* ('cover-up') seems to avoid the practice of informing the broader population about the existing problems. Perhaps this principle is related not only to professional mistakes, but also to the gaps in the system, as we observed a lot of socially desirable answers in our study. Indeed, when general questions were asked (whether there is a job appraisal system, whether it works well), respondents provided an answer which describes the practices in a positive way, but further detailed questions bring less positive insights of the system organisation and practices to light.

Monetary motivation may play an important role in rewarding professional behaviour, but formally, chief doctors have little financial autonomy or available resources. When they are available, financial bonuses are traditionally used to reward long-term work at the facility or an anniversary (for instance, one of the respondents stated that staff in their facility get bonuses at 50-year anniversaries). Despite little opportunity to provide monetary incentives, there are some informal methods to reward the personnel: for instance, opportunity to take a day off, flexibility in choosing vacation periods and issuing letters of recognition are used as informal stimuli by facility management.

In a nutshell, the system of performance appraisal that exists at the time of this study does not seem to be designed with regard to the key goal of stimulating professional development. By contrast, it is focused on punishment for bad performance, rather than a reward for good practices at the hospital. Financial motivation for good performance is almost non-existent, while non-financial motivation (not punishment) is rarely used.

Discussion and conclusions

By and large, the performance of healthcare providers under the governmental financial and regulatory framework is virtually unconnected with the formal system of incentives (financial as well as other less tangible incentives). Still, healthcare providers – having a salary lower than the industrial average – are expected not only to demonstrate professional behaviour, but also to generate funds for the facility to which they belong.

Our ethnographical explorative study has some limitations. The results should not be taken as representative given the lack of comparativeness between regions as well as between medical specialities, a relatively small sample and convenient sample technique. The extensive mode of data collection and combination of closed- and open-ended questions may have confused some of the respondents and caused differences in coding their answers. Upon the agreement of respondents, all the interviews are recorded on audio, which possibly could have lowered their willingness to respond to sensitive questions. Despite the limitations mentioned, the study offers a description of the mix of formal–informal practices at state healthcare facilities which have to be overcome for the improvement of the professional behaviour of medical staff.

More power in the healthcare market, or informational asymmetry, coupled with access to patient payments, encourages Ukrainian physicians to act as both fund recipients and brokers, intermediaries between holders of funds (patients) and managers of the funds (healthcare facilities). The study results suggest that informal patient payments given to healthcare service providers are partially passed to department heads or chief doctors and further (Belli *et al.*, 2015).

When the system of bonuses is weak but 'envelope' payments are major incentives for providers (a higher weight for informal rather than formal stimuli), it brings a lot of ambiguity to the system of healthcare service provision. At the moment in Ukraine, patients' feedback (financially or via marketing buzz) on doctors' performance plays a major role in stimulating professionalism. Shishkin and colleagues (2003, p. 29), for example, describe two strategies used by young doctors in terms of professionalism: some 'are trying to compensate the lack of professionalism by actively extorting money from patients (at any price)', while others improve their professional knowledge, skills and experience 'in order to obtain the same unspoken right to charge for services, as more experienced doctors have'. Still, when the informal economy prevails in the sector with an interwoven lack of restraints and disrespect for law, it is also threatened with the loss of morality of medical doctors and, therefore, the loss of professionalism in general (Bazylevych, 2009).

Very similar barriers to the enhancement of professionalism are found in post-Soviet Lithuania: an unexpected link to informal payments related to the topic of professional growth has been discovered where salaries and work conditions have been sheltered and controlled by the state (Riska and Novelskaite, 2011). The authors also conclude that 'in a post-socialist health care system, physicians are often operating in a system guided by four logics: the state, the market, professional culture, and the informal economy of peer referrals, gift giving, and extra payments' (Riska and Novelskaite, 2011, p. 89).

Nevertheless, informal practices are sensitive to politics, as the case of Cambodia also shows: the formalisation of the under-the-counter payments has been designed as the first step toward the growth of professionalism (Dieleman and Harnmeijer, 2006). The country offers an example of a transformation that has displayed positive effects on professionalism in healthcare after new policy implementation. In particular, the introduction of flat fees has brought not only clear patients' and providers' roles and responsibilities, but also financial resources to healthcare facilities obtained via official channels that make possible the introduction of performance-related bonus systems (Barber, Bonnet and Bekedam, 2004; Dieleman and Harnmeijer, 2006). Although a performance-related system might bring controversy to the value system of a profession where altruism opposes incentivising performance (Buurman and Dur, 2012; Lindkvist, 2013), Cambodia has made a step not only toward a more civilised system of provider payments, but also toward consumerism and the market orientation of healthcare services, which bring new approaches for ensuring professionalism and the role of altruism.

Furthermore, evidence-based practices have become an important push–factor in the development of the medical profession connected with 'software' or processes–related changes in healthcare provision (McKinlay and Marceau, 2008; Timmermanns and Oh, 2010). Indeed, the design and implementation of a system of stimuli, in which additional educational activities are supported by the facility administration, and measures are taken to make the market of vacancies more transparent, does not require large resources but, rather, good managerial skills and knowledge of best practices. Patients' complaints or feedback, for example, are rarely taken into account in decision–making, possibly because of lack of knowledge and applicable tools in the field. Good managerial practice is even more important in the context of limited resources as it does not require additional funds (as in the case of buying new modern equipment).

Moreover, our study reveals that other sources to fund participation in external events are provided by pharmaceutical companies, but one should consider possible bias toward the company products, which might not be the most effective and cost–efficient. There should be clear guidelines and policies which ensure ethics in public sector and pharmaceutical industry collaboration (Relman, 2001).

As has also been mentioned above, professionalism is rated as the fourth most problematic issue in Romanian healthcare after corruption, lack of modern equipment and lack of interest of medical staff. However, all three top-rated dimensions contribute to medical professionalism: attention and good attitude toward patients, the utilisation of safety technologies and modern equipment, and transparency in service provision are integral parts of healthcare profession–alism. Moreover, lack of practices which are conducted in line with morality and an ethical code affects trust in state medical and healthcare institutions (Blumenthal, 1994). Lack of professionalism and trust may turn up in the most responsible and unexpected moments. For example, it was especially problem–atic during the Maidan clashes in 2014 in Ukraine when patients with trauma avoided state emergency service providers and searched for voluntary medical care (Stepurko *et al.*, 2014).

Healthcare systems with very limited resources are expected to find creative and 'soft' decisions when good health outcomes are in the political agenda. Meanwhile, a lack of political will to confront poor performance of service providers, harmful practices and inappropriate care is often observed when an institution's effectiveness is undermined 'by diverting it from its purpose or weakening its ability to achieve its purpose' (so–called 'institutional corruption') (Lessig, 2013, p. 553).

Swick (2000) emphasises the embeddedness of the medical profession in social and family life, as well as the importance of relationships between patient and physician. In line with this, the context of most post-Soviet societies can be described as lower state control of public services after the collapse of the Soviet Union, changes in the roles of institutions, slow pace of democratic and market-led reforms, as well as 'the self-serving authorities against a poor and defenceless population' (Wanner, 2005; Sanghera and Iliasov, 2008; Riska and Novelskaite, 2011). Following the general trend, not only the medical profession, its ethics and morale, but also the general understanding of professionalism has been constructed under a new reality, values and norms. As Sanghera and Iliasov (2008, p. 3) argue, 'professions in post-socialist societies emphasize the relationship between the state and the professions in terms of control and discipline, suggesting that professionals lack the critical autonomy and integrity necessary to shape their social field'. Therefore, the challenge of finding the balance between economic restraints, cultural context, and work autonomy and identity is faced by many professions in post-Soviet environments, especially those who are salaried and strongly controlled by the state.

To summarise, multiple barriers exist to the enforcement of healthcare professionalism in Ukraine. The importance of personal connections does not contribute to transparency in appointments or the discovery and prevention of bad practices in healthcare and the stimulating of good ones, and, therefore, it threatens the health outcomes and attributes of healthcare services. Human resources, as the most important resource in the healthcare sector, require proper managerial practices framed by relevant and respectful regulations in order to ensure adequate access to and quality of healthcare services.

Acknowledgements

This research was undertaken with support from the World Bank. The content of the publication is the sole responsibility of the authors and in no way represents the views of the World Bank. We would like to acknowledge the great contribution of the organisations which implemented the study: FISCO ID (Yuriy Dzhygyr, Kateryna Maynzyuk) and Kyiv International Institute of Sociology (a team of researchers and interviewers under the supervision of Artem Myroshnychenko). We are grateful to the medical doctors, nurses, healthcare managers and decision-makers who agreed to participate in our study. We appreciate the support of our colleagues and research team who facilitated the carrying out of this research and without whose participation this research would have been impossible.

Note

1 According to Transparency International (2014), Ukraine ranked 142 out of 175 countries, and low rates of political stability are observed in the Worldwide Governance Indicators (2013), which rank Ukraine at 21.3 in contrast to Poland at 78.7 or Belarus at 46.4. Health expenditure per capita is currently equal to US$313 and public health expenditure stands at 54.5 per cent of total health expenditure (WHO Global Health Observatory Data Repository, 2013).

References

Barber, S., Bonnet, F. and Bekedam, H., 2004. Formalizing under-the-table payments to control out-of-pocket hospital expenditures in Cambodia. *Health Policy and Planning*, 19(4), pp. 199–208.

Bazylevych, M., 2009. Who is responsible for our health? Changing concepts of state and the individual in post-soviet Ukraine. *Anthropology of East Europe Review*, 27(1), pp. 65–75.

Belli, P., Dzygyr, Y. and Maynzyuk, K., 2015. *How is it working? A new approach to measure governance in the health care system in Ukraine.* The World Bank: Obnova Company. Available through: <http://cop.health-rights.org/files/f/8/f82ced28c2386b 53adf34ee54d80c1fe.pdf> [accessed on 13 August 2015].

Blumenthal, D., 1994. The vital role of professionalism in health care reform. *Health Affairs*, 13(1), pp. 252–6.

Buurman, M. and Dur, R., 2012. Incentives and the sorting of altruistic agents into street-level bureaucracies. *Scandinavian Journal of Economics*, 114(4), pp. 1318–45.

Chisholm, M.A., Cobb, H., Duke, L., McDuffie, C. and Kennedy, W.K., 2006. Development of an instrument to measure professionalism. *American Journal of Pharmaceutical Education*, 70(4), p. 85.

Danyliv, A., Stepurko, T., Gryga, I., Pavlova, M. and Groot, W., 2012. Is there a place for the patient in the Ukrainian health care system? Patient payment policies and investment priorities in health care in Ukraine. *Society and Economy*, 34(2), pp. 273–91.

Dieleman, M. and Harnmeijer, J.W., 2006. *Improving health worker performance: in search of promising practices.* Geneva: World Health Organization, pp. 5–34.

Fărcăşanu, D., 2010. Population perception on corruption, informal payments and introduction of co-payments in the public health system in Romania. *Management in Health*, 14(1), pp. 8–13.

Gryga, I., Stepurko, T., Danyliv, A., Gryga, M., Lynnyk, O., Pavlova, M. and Groot, W., 2010. Attitudes towards patient payments in Ukraine: is there a place for official patient charges. *Zeszyty Naukowe Ochrony Zdrowia. Zdrowie Publiczne I Zarzadzanie*, 13(1), pp. 69–78.

Ledeneva, A.V., 1998. *Russia's economy of favours: Blat, networking and informal exchange.* Cambridge: Cambridge University Press.

Lekhan, V., Rudiy, V., Shevchenko, M., Nitzan, K.D. and Richardson, E., 2015. Ukraine: health system review. *Health Systems in Transition*, 17(2), pp. 1–154.

Lessig, L., 2013. Institutional corruption defined. *Journal of Law, Medicine and Ethics*, 41, pp. 553–5.

Lindkvist, I., 2013. Informal payments and health worker effort: a quantitative study from Tanzania. *Health Economics*, 22(10), pp. 1250–71.

McKinlay, J.B. and Marceau, L.D., 2008. When there is no doctor: reasons for the disappearance of primary care physicians in the US during the early 21st century. *Social Science and Medicine*, 67, pp. 1481–91.

Passi, V., Doug, M., Peile, J.T. and Johnson, N., 2010. Developing medical professionalism in future doctors: a systematic review. *International Journal of Medical Education*, 1, pp. 19–29.

Pavlova, M., Tambor, M., Stepurko, T., van Merode, G.G. and Groot, W. (2012). Assessment of patient payment policy in CEE countries: from a conceptual framework to policy indicators. *Society and Economy*, 34(2), pp. 193–220.

Polese, A., 2014. Informal payments in Ukrainian hospitals: on the boundary between informal payments, gifts, and bribes. *Anthropological Forum*, 24(4), pp. 381–95.

Polese, A. and Stepurko, T., 2016. Ukraine – 2016: where is the state? Web blog post at Ukrainska pravda; in Ukrainian, March 10. Available through: <www.pravda.com.ua/rus/columns/2016/03/10/7101463/?attempt=1> [accessed on 1 April 2016].

Rechel, B. and McKee, M., 2009. Health reform in central and eastern Europe and the former Soviet Union. *Lancet*, 374, pp. 1186–95.

Relman, A.S., 2001. Separating continuing medical education from pharmaceutical marketing. *JAMA*, 285(15), pp. 2009–12.

Riska, E. and Novelskaite, A., 2011. Professionalism and medical work in a post-Soviet society: between four logics. *Anthropology of East Europe Review*, 29(1), pp. 82–93.

Sanghera, B. and Iliasov, A., 2008. Moral sentiments and professionalism in post-Soviet Kyrgyzstan: understanding professional practices and ethics. *International Sociology*, 23(3), pp. 447–67.

Shishkin, S., Bogatova, T., Potapchik, Y., Chernets, V., Chirikova, A. and Shilova, L., 2003. *Informal out-of-pocket payments for healthcare in Russia*. Moscow: Independent Institute for Social Policy.

Stepurko, T., Pavlova, M., Gryga, I. and Groot, W., 2013. Informal payments for health care services – corruption or gratitude? A study on public attitudes, perceptions and opinions in six central and eastern European countries. *Communist and Post-Communist Studies*, 46(4), pp. 419–31.

Stepurko, T., Vitiuk, V., Kvit, A. and Kovtonyuk, P., 2014. Medical care on the Euromaidan: who have saved the lives of the protesters? *Social, Health, and Communication Studies Journal*, 1(1), pp. 80–104.

Swick, H.M. 2000. Toward a normative definition of medical professionalism. *Academic Medicine*, 75, pp. 612–16.

Tambor, M., Pavlova, M., Rechel, B., Golinowska, S., Sowada, C. and Groot, W., 2014. The inability to pay for health services in Central and Eastern Europe: evidence from six countries. *European Journal of Public Health*, 24(3), pp. 378–85.

Timmermanns, S. and Oh, H., 2010. The continued social transformation of the medical profession. *Journal of Health and Social Behavior*, 51, pp. 94–106.

Tourangeau, R. and Smith, T.W., 1996. Asking sensitive questions: the impact of data collection mode, question format, and question context. *Public Opinion Quarterly*, 60(2), pp. 275–304.

Transparency International, 2014. Corruption perception index 2014. Available through: <www.transparency.org/country#UKR> [accessed on 14 August 2015].

Veloski, J.J., Fields, S.K., Boex, J.R. and Blank, L.L., 2005. Measuring professionalism: a review of studies with instruments reported in the literature between 1982 and 2002. *Academic Medicine*, 80(4), pp. 366–70.

Wanner, C., 2005. Money, morality and new forms of exchange in postsocialist Ukraine. *Ethnos*, 70(4), pp. 515–37.

WHO Global Health Observatory Data Repository, 2013. Available through: <http://apps.who.int/gho/data/view.main.680> [accessed on 14 August 2015].

Williams, C.C. and Onoschenko, O., 2013. The diverse livelihood practices of healthcare workers in Ukraine. In: J. Morris and A. Polese eds., *The informal post-socialist economy: embedded practices and livelihoods*. New York: Routledge, Ch. 1.

Worldwide Governance Indicators, 2013. Political stability and absence of violence. Available through: <http://info.worldbank.org/governance/wgi/index.aspx#country Reports> [accessed on 14 August 2015].

7 Transformation of the role of healthcare ethics committees and the concept of clinical ethics in Belarus

Implications for medical professionalism

Andrei Famenka

Introduction

Professionalism in medicine has attracted considerable attention in recent years and has been seen increasingly as a significant issue for the current state and future prospects of medicine (Wynia *et al.*, 1999). One reason for this is the concern that healthcare professionals as a social group will gradually lose their distinctive voice in public debate about healthcare, which is progressively dominated by economic and other corporate interests (Swick, 1998). In this debate, physicians are usually associated with the role of experts, whose task is limited to applying their skills and knowledge to the process of healing. However, this narrow view of medical professionalism tends to ignore the important public and social purposes served by the medical profession.

In this chapter, the role of the professional ethics of physicians in strengthening medical professionalism and restoring the social weight of the medical profession is discussed. Clinical ethics consultation (CEC) is presented as an example of an appropriate vehicle for promoting medical professionalism and accomplishing the task of providing ethical support to healthcare professionals in a time of moral uncertainty. For the purpose of this chapter, the situation concerning CEC in Belarus is used as a case study example to illustrate the importance of the context for CEC development and its influence on medical professionalism. A number of factors of sociopolitical and economic post-communist transition in Belarus are shown as playing key roles in making the environment in which CEC services operate adversarial to ethical reflection and democratisation. The discussion focuses on the negative consequences of the adoption of a misleading concept of clinical ethics in Belarus and the established practice of forcing physicians to adhere to professional norms. It is argued that the notion of professionalism in Belarus is used as a means of exercising control over the medical profession for the sake of certain societal and political interests. The chapter ends with the conclusion that the underlying causes of the misuse of CEC services in Belarus are tightly linked with the developmental factors of post-communist transition. It is also emphasised that the presence of societal and political conditions affirmative to ethical reflection and democratisation in healthcare, and in society as a whole, is crucial for ensuring the proper functioning of CEC services and successful promotion of medical professionalism.

An appropriate account of medical professionalism

It has been recognised since ancient times that a special set of responsibilities to patients constitutes an essential element of the identity of healthcare professionals and provides a necessary basis for establishing relations of trust between patients and physicians. However, a recent trend of shifting the focus of attention from the moral foundations of the medical profession to the scope and content of medical interventions makes it harder to discern the very basic imperative of healthcare professionals to serve the best interests of patients and promote their wellbeing. Arguably, an excessive focus on the expert knowledge of physicians is likely to have a negative impact not only on their social status, but also on their own self-identification as a professional group (Kovács, 2010). Thus, an appropriate account of medical professionalism should rest upon a combination of scientific knowledge, technical skills and professional ethics of physicians. This integrative view of medical professionalism corresponds with the social function of the medical profession, and can serve as a driving force for promoting professional integrity and restoring medicine's distinctive voice in public debate.

There have been several attempts to elaborate on the holistic account of medical professionalism and conceptualise it in such a way that it would be broad enough to incorporate all of its basic dimensions and, at the same time, be sufficiently detailed to guide healthcare professionals through the complex environment of contemporary medical practice. One prominent example of this kind is the 'Medical professionalism in the new millennium: a physician charter', developed by the American Board of Internal Medicine, the American College of Physicians and the European Federation of Internal Medicine (ABIM, 2002). This charter takes a holistic approach to the issue of medical professionalism by encompassing a set of fundamental principles and relevant commitments. The charter incorporates three principles: the primacy of patient welfare, patient autonomy and social justice. It also contains a set of specific commitments, including improving access to high-quality healthcare, advocating for a just distribution of finite resources and managing conflicts of interest. The same holistic approach, but with a greater emphasis on the behavioural aspects of practising the medical profession, has been used by Swick (2000) in his attempt to develop a normative definition of medical professionalism. Swick proposes a set of behaviours that constitute medical professionalism, and that healthcare professionals are supposed to demonstrate if they are to remain trustworthy in the eyes of patients and preserve their integrity as a professional group. An important point, which is underscored both in the charter on medical professionalism and in its normative account, is that healthcare professionals must fully comprehend what medical professionalism entails. That is, by embracing the comprehensive view on medical professionalism, physicians demonstrate the commitment to meet the demands and expectations aroused among patients, colleagues and broader society in response to this account of professionalism.

However, as appropriate as these conceptualisations of medical professionalism are, they lack a clear vision for translating theoretical considerations into practice. This is especially true with regard to the ethical component of medical professionalism, which is far more difficult to teach and cultivate than technical skills and scientific knowledge. Given that the nature of healthcare professionals' work and the environments in which they operate are becoming increasingly complex, physicians might not be well-prepared to adapt themselves to these rapid changes. Additionally, in an era of plurality of values, physicians might feel that they lack the necessary expertise, skills and knowledge to solve the moral dilemmas raised by the recent advancements of biotechnology and medical science.

Clinical ethics consultation as a vehicle for promoting medical professionalism

The complexity of the contemporary clinical environment and the challenges it might generate for physicians are compelling arguments to claim that the ethical component of medical professionalism needs special attention and effective support. One suggestion about how this support might be provided is to bring medical ethics closer to clinical practice by implementing special services and structures offering ethical assistance to healthcare professionals (Yen and Schneiderman, 1999). The idea is to make medical ethics more practically oriented by using it for identifying, analysing and solving ethical problems that arise in contemporary healthcare. In order to achieve this objective, a range of approaches to provide CEC – a generic term for different kinds of ethical support services – has been suggested, developed and implemented worldwide in recent years; healthcare ethics committees (HECs) and ethics consultation (EC) are the most notable examples of these. With regard to medical professionalism, it has been argued that CEC might be useful in its promotion both at the organisational level, by helping to clarify ethical values of an institution and place them at the centre of a hospital's mission, and at the individual level, by serving as a platform for reflections on professional values and norms through the lens of individual clinical cases (Kovács, 2010). In general, it has been expected that CEC would facilitate reflections on how the ethical component of medical professionalism could be revitalised and adapted to the contemporary clinical environment in a time when the foundations of professional norms in medicine are challenged by economic and other corporate interests (Stüber, 2010).

However, the positive effect on medical professionalism can only be achieved if CEC structures are implemented and maintained in a way that does not contradict the general purposes of clinical ethics: to educate, serve and provide policy analysis regarding ethical problems arising in clinical settings (Siegler, Pellegrino and Singer, 1990). In recent years, clinical ethics has also been increasingly conceived as a vehicle for the promotion of biomedical citizenship and democratisation in healthcare (Lebeer, 2005). Within this framework, the main purposes of CEC services can be defined as facilitating and practising moral deliberation in institutional healthcare delivery. Ascribing CEC structures with tasks other than these could, therefore, conflict with the core functions of CECs and might prevent them from doing their job properly. It appears that the misuse of CEC services could simply make the task of providing healthcare professionals with appropriate ethical support unrealisable in practice. Moreover, this misuse might be detrimental to the idea of strengthening the ethical component of medical professionalism and to efforts aimed at revitalising the fundamental ethical principles of the medical profession.

However, examples of the misuse of CEC services are not rare. A paradigmatic example of this kind, described in studies on the development and maintenance of CEC services, is the use of these structures for the sake of crisis management and conflict resolution (Beyleveld, Brownsword and Wallace, 2002; Steinkamp *et al.*, 2007). Other examples of the misuse of CEC services include assigning them with the task of reviewing protocols of biomedical studies, that is, to deal with research ethics, which is conceptually and methodologically different from clinical ethics (Meulenbergs, Vermylen and Schotsmans, 2005; Borovećki, ten Have and Orešković, 2005). The phenomenon of the misuse of CEC services requires serious attention, as it might be indicative of the conceptual assumptions which underlie the goals and purposes of CEC and actual perceptions about medical professionalism.

Clinical ethics consultation services in context: framework for assessment

Although CEC services operate mainly at the institutional level, the processes of their establishment and maintenance are influenced not only by special features of a host organisation, but also by the factors of broader societal, political and economic origin (Vollmann, 2010). In this regard, exploring the environment in which the impact of the latter factors is substantial can be helpful for emphasising the importance of the broader context for CEC development and maintenance. For these purposes, the situation regarding CEC services in Belarus is used as a case study example of the misuse of CEC services, with the aim of shedding light on the role that contextual factors play in shaping perceptions about clinical ethics and medical professionalism. The case can be of interest for both a national and an international readership, as it illustrates a number of barriers to the effective functioning of CEC services. Given that there have only been a few attempts to provide a systematic analysis of the broader contextual conditions and their effect on the performance of CEC (Gefenas, 2001; Borovećki *et al.*, 2005), this case analysis provides an opportunity to explore further the ways and mechanisms by which broader political and societal factors shape the way in which CEC services are established and maintained.

However, in the absence of a coherent conceptual framework for assessing CEC services, attempts to identify the impact that contextual conditions have on the actual functioning and current practices of CEC might be challenging and problematic. One way of overcoming these difficulties might be to adapt a framework developed for similar purposes and applied to the structures having relevant goals and similar characteristics. For the purposes of this chapter, the framework for assessing research ethics systems suggested by Hyder *et al.* (2009) and based on Sen's model of development as freedom (1999) has been suggested for use as an analytical platform. The main idea behind this framework is that the basic freedoms that Sen (1999) describes as being constitutive of development are necessary foundations for any research ethics system. In this model, the research ethics review function is systemically linked to: (1) national and regional strategies (e.g. legal and regulatory authority for research ethics committees, national guidelines, budget priority for research ethics, investment in training and capacity building); (2) institutional commitment (e.g. organisational structures and procedures, conformity with national and regional laws and guidance); (3) research ethics review characteristics (independence of research ethics committees, scrutiny of review, procedural clarity and consistency of decisions); and (4) researcher's conduct (e.g. respect for government, institution, committee). Surrounding these systems are (5) enabling conditions, such as strong civil society, public accountability and trust in basic transactional processes. In turn, these are surrounded by (6) development conditions, including political freedoms, economic facilities, social opportunities and transparency guarantees. According to the view of Hyder and colleagues (2009), this larger context within which the research ethics system operates is a key determinant of its performance. Similarly, CEC services can be conceptualised as a vehicle for facilitating ethical reflection in clinical settings, which does not proceed in a vacuum, but in a complex environment with certain political, societal, economic and cultural characteristics, all of which are likely to make an impact on the shape and functions of CEC services. Drawing on these conceptual assumptions, the Hyder *et al.* (2009) framework has been adapted to the needs of CEC assessment and applied to CEC services in Belarus.

Clinical ethics consultation services in Belarus: aiming at the wrong target

CEC is a relatively new phenomenon in Belarus. The development of CEC services as a systematic process began in the late-1990s when the regulatory framework for clinical ethics was officially introduced at the level of a national healthcare system (Ministry of Health of the Republic of Belarus, 1999). This move was preceded by the development and promulgation of the 'Code of medical ethics' in 1999, which was a product of a series of discussions within the medical profession during several conferences and meetings at the national level (Belarusian Medical Association, 1999). In contrast to the majority of Western European countries where basic elements of CEC have been developing in a 'grass roots' fashion (Steinkamp *et al.*, 2007), in Belarus, the system of CEC has been implemented through a quite rigorous 'top-down' approach. This move represented tremendous progress in the development of clinical ethics in Belarus, given that prior to that move, there were no officially documented ethical consultations taking place in Belarus. Thus, due to this official recognition, a regulatory framework for the development and functioning of CEC has been set up. It has been chosen as the way to run an HEC model of clinical ethics support in Belarus. This means that EC is supposed to be provided on a non-professional basis by a team of dedicated hospital employees for whom this activity constitutes a part of their multifaceted clinical jobs. At that time, regulation of HECs in Belarus was decentralised and rather weak. However, after only a few years, new regulations have come into force and brought about changes in terms of the scope and content of the work of HECs and characteristics of the regulations themselves. The establishment of HECs in medical facilities has become a requirement which was introduced by the amended version of the Law on the Healthcare System in 2008 (NRLRB, 2008). Regulation of HECs has also become centralised and strict. The National Medical Ethics Committee has been established and charged with the task, *inter alia*, of coordinating and overseeing the activity of all HECs in the country (Ministry of Health of the Republic of Belarus, 2006). In fact, these amendments and their implications merit serious attention, since at least some of them deviate significantly from what is considered to be the core mission and general purpose of HECs. The amendments give rise to justifiable concerns with regard to the abilities of these reshaped HECs to perform their main function, i.e. to facilitate ethical reflection in healthcare settings. Although the reasons behind the decision of the health authorities to transform HECs have never been clearly articulated and openly conveyed to the public, an analysis of the political, economic and social environment in terms of the Hyder *et al.* (2009) framework can help one understand the root causes of this turn of events.

Developmental conditions constitute the first of the six domains in the adapted framework. Belarus is a former Soviet Union republic which became independent in 1991. The most striking difference between Belarus and its neighbouring countries is that after the breakdown of the Soviet Union and collapse of the Eastern Bloc, Belarus decided not to follow the path leading to adoption of the European criteria on democracy and the rule of law. In contrast to the Baltic countries, Poland and other Eastern European neighbours, Belarus has developed differently. After independence, the political environment in Belarus deteriorated significantly (CEPA and Freedom House, 2011). Two years after the first presidential elections in 1994, the country was downgraded to the 'Not Free' category in Freedom House's annual 'Freedom in the World' survey. To this day, Belarus still remains in the category 'World's Most Repressive Societies' (Freedom House, 2013). Belarus constantly faces criticism from international bodies on the grounds of perceived unfair elections and violations of human rights, restrictions of the freedom of expression, lack of independence of judiciary and pressure on civil society (OSCE/ODIHR, 2010). The pace of economic reform in Belarus has been evolutionary and moderate (UNDP, 2005). According to the data of The World Bank (2015), Belarus is one of the least reformed countries in the region. The Transparency International (2014) Corruption Perceptions Index score for Belarus is 31 compared to 58 for neighbouring Lithuania on a scale from 0 (highly corrupt) to 100 (very clean).

The second domain in the adapted framework involves the enabling conditions. In Belarus, like in many other 'transitional' countries of Central and Eastern Europe, the turbulent period of radical political and economic changes has significantly influenced the ethical climate of society and has led to ambiguity and vagueness of the prevalent moral norms (Tichtchenko and Yudin, 1997). Newly adopted laws have proved unable to change the patterns of people's behaviour immediately, despite their rhetoric to do so (Jakusovaite and Bankauskaite, 2007). Thus, as Silis (2010) points out, current moral standards in transitional countries might well be conceived as those representing an odd mixture of not yet rooted new values and not yet extinguished old traditions. With regard to the power of civil society and effectiveness of mechanisms of public participation, the lack of these two is typical for countries in the region, including Belarus. The current organisational structure of the healthcare system in Belarus is quite rigid and highly centralised, and does not facilitate public participation (Richardson *et al.*, 2013). In addition, communities themselves are weak because of lack of cohesion, democratic culture and traditions of public participation (Dryzek and Holmes, 2002).

Enabling conditions give rise to the third domain in the adapted framework – a national and regional strategy for CEC. As outlined above, the establishment of HECs in Belarusian healthcare facilities is required by the Law on the Healthcare System of the Republic of Belarus (NRLRB, 2008). The issues related to the mission, tasks, structure and processes of HECs are further defined in the ministerial guidelines on that matter. The current type of regulation of HECs can be characterised as strict and centralised, whereas previous regulatory documents have been oriented towards a rather weak and decentralised approach to the regulation of HECs. An early regulatory document, the 'Model Guidelines for Healthcare Ethics Committees' was issued by the Ministry of Health of Belarus in 1999 and delineated the function of HECs as being aimed at increasing and promoting knowledge of medical ethics among healthcare practitioners, analysing and solving ethical problems arising in day-to-day clinical practice, making recommendations and developing appropriate strategies to tackle these ethical problems (Ministry of Health of the Republic of Belarus, 1999). Thus, HECs at that time were conceived as consultative rather than disciplinary bodies.

New regulations on HECs came into force in 2006 and assigned HECs with a new set of responsibilities, primarily concerned with the resolution of conflicts between healthcare professionals and patients, and among healthcare professionals themselves. The HECs have also been ascribed the task of monitoring healthcare professionals' adherence to professional norms and institutional codes of conduct. Under these regulations, HECs have been given the right to recommend that local health authorities impose disciplinary sanctions on healthcare professionals (Ministry of Health of the Republic of Belarus, 2006). The National Medical Ethics Committee has been established as a coordinating body for all HECs in the country, and has been supposed to serve as a body of appeal and review of HECs' statements and opinions upon request (Ministry of Health of the Republic of Belarus, 2006). The reasons behind this change can be found in the preamble of the decree on the establishment of The National Medical Ethics Committee: 'in order to effectively ensure the implementation of the Presidential decrees and the Council of Ministers' ordinances on handling of citizens' complaints', meaning that HECs have become regarded merely as a tool for performing administrative procedures and promoting the views of those with political power.

Institutional commitment constitutes the fourth domain in the adapted framework. According to Hyder *et al.* (2009), the priority that institutions give to the responsibility for ethical review (in the adapted framework it equates to the notion of CEC) can be judged by the appropriateness of the structures and procedures for review (again, it equates to the notion of CEC in the adapted framework) and emphasis on ethical conduct within the institution. On the institutional level this commitment provides a basis for the fifth domain of the framework, i.e. safeguarding the independence of research ethics committees from undue bias and promoting the quality of the scrutiny and the consistency of judgement. However, due to the lack of direct, comprehensive and reliable information, these domains can currently be described only by making inferences from the laws, guidelines and statutes pertaining to HECs in Belarus. With regard to the CEC structures, the 'Model Guidelines for Healthcare Ethics Committees' provides the requirements on the membership and composition of HECs, stating that an HEC has to be composed of no fewer than five members, all of whom should be healthcare professionals working in the institution that establishes the HEC (Ministry of Health of the Republic of Belarus, 2008). No specific requirements have been put forward with regard to the qualifications, background, age and gender of the members. Additionally, the 'Model Guidelines for Healthcare Ethics Committees' does not contain formal requirements with regard to initial training and ongoing education for the HEC members (Ministry of Health of the Republic of Belarus, 2008). The only legally recognised inclusive criterion for potential HEC members is that they belong to a specific professional medical group, since formally no expertise in clinical ethics was required. The practical work on the committee is the main method of acquiring appropriate competence for HEC members. It should be noted, however, that the basic knowledge of clinical ethics among healthcare professionals in Belarus, which could be regarded as a foundation for developing practical skills on CEC, is absolutely insufficient, because of the extremely low attention paid to bioethics at the undergraduate and postgraduate levels of medical education (Kubar, 2010).

The final domain in the adapted framework is that of a physician's conduct (in the original version – investigator's conduct). Unfortunately, no research has been performed in Belarus on the aspects of a physician's conduct in terms of medical professionalism, therefore, this domain can only be outlined in very general terms and presented as a product of other elements in the model. It been argued that CEC might be useful in the promotion of medical professionalism, by serving as a platform for reflections on professional values and norms through the lens of individual clinical cases (Kovács, 2010). In this regard, a question might be raised concerning the ability of HECs in Belarus to facilitate ethical reflection and democratic deliberation in the healthcare settings, given their recent transformation into the sort of disciplinary bodies and promoters of values imposed from above. Ascribing to HECs the authority to solve conflicts and render disciplinary sanctions has effectively shaped HECs to the point where ethics support has been pushed to the margins of their activities.

The case of the transformation of HECs in Belarus cannot be explained by referring only to the specific characteristics of organisations that establish HECs, without paying considerable attention to the political and socio-economic conditions in which healthcare organisations and HECs operate. In this regard, the situation in Belarus corresponds with the bureaucratic approach to the establishment of a system of CEC observed in some other countries of Central and Eastern Europe (Gefenas, 2001; Borovečki *et al.*, 2005). It has been argued that this tendency stems from the common Soviet legacy of an authoritarian style of regulation covering every aspect of social life, including healthcare. Belarus has inherited a lot from the Soviet times, therefore, the domestic variation of the establishment of CEC services leading to a transformation of HECs into disciplinary panels could be the result of a preservation of the traditional dominance of interests of the state over individual rights of its citizens. In these conditions, an authoritarian, non–deliberative concept of medical and clinical ethics prevails. For those who have adopted the misleading concept of medical ethics, forcing physicians to adhere to professional norms constitutes not only an acceptable, but also the preferable way to promote medical professionalism. However, in reality, the use of HECs in the form of disciplinary panels effectively limits the autonomy of the medical profession and, therefore, diminishes the social status of healthcare professionals. The idea of strengthening the ethical component of medical professionalism through the promotion of CEC services is likely to become compromised, and the efforts supposed to be aimed at revitalising fundamental professional principles appear to move in completely the opposite direction. As a result of this move, the

medical profession has become more dependent on certain political and economic interests than before. On the practical level, ascribing CEC structures
with tasks other than those relevant to their core mission effectively prevents
them from being really beneficial for healthcare professionals in terms of providing support in a time of moral uncertainty. The case of the implementation
of CEC services in Belarus shows that adoption of a misleading concept of
clinical ethics produces only counterproductive results, because, in the eyes
of healthcare professionals, Belarusian HECs have become opponents rather
than supporters and allies.

Conclusion

The analysis of the implementation of CEC services in Belarus shows that the
development and maintenance of CEC services are tightly linked with broader
sociopolitical and economic frameworks, which, in the case of Belarus, constitute a set of factors of post-communist transition. These factors are, at least in
part, responsible for making the environment in which CEC services operate
adversarial to ethical reflection and democratisation. Transformation of the
HEC into a sort of disciplinary panel impacts the ethical component of medical
professionalism negatively and diminishes the value of the internal commitment of healthcare professionals to serve the best interests of the patients and
promote their wellbeing. This, in turn, weakens the healthcare professionals'
confidence in the power of their professional integrity.

The practice of forcing physicians to adhere to their professional norms
limits the autonomy of the medical profession and impacts on the social status
of healthcare professionals negatively. In the misleading concept of medical
ethics, the notion of professionalism is used as a means to exercise control over
the medical profession for the sake of certain societal and political interests.

The example of Belarus suggests that, in the absence of development and
enabling conditions for CEC services, there is a danger that any system for
facilitating ethical reflection in healthcare settings, irrespective of how promising its starting position might be, is likely to be misused. There is a need for
more research to be performed on the issues of CEC and medical professionalism. Making the underlying causes of the misuse of CEC services clear is an
important task which should be accomplished not only to ensure the proper
functioning of the CEC, but also to promote medical professionalism that is
free from external influence and serves the interests of patients, healthcare
professionals and society in general.

References

ABIM: American Board of Internal Medicine Foundation, American College of
Physicians Foundation and European Federation of Internal Medicine, 2002.
Medical professionalism in the new millennium: a physician charter. *Annals of Internal
Medicine*, 136, pp. 243–6.

Belarusian Medical Association, 1999. *Code of medical ethics (in Russian)*. Available through: www.beldoc.by/documents/2a6db062a0f6cf1d23523dd295eedc5f/ [accessed 31 August 2015].

Beyleveld, D., Brownsword, R. and Wallace, S., 2002. Clinical Ethics Committees: clinician support or crisis management? *HEC Forum*, 14(1), pp. 13–25.

Borovećki, A., ten Have, H., Orešković, S., 2005. Ethics and the structures of health care in the European countries in transition: hospital ethics committees in Croatia. *British Medical Journal*, 331, pp. 227–9.

CEPA: Centre for European Policy Analysis and Freedom House, 2011. *Democratic change in Belarus: a framework for action*. Available through: <https://freedomhouse. org/event/democratic-change-belarus-framework-action> [accessed 27 August 2015].

Dryzek, J.S. and Holmes, L.T., 2002. *Post-communist democratization: political discourses across thirteen countries*. Cambridge: Cambridge University Press.

Freedom House, 2013. *Freedom in the world: democratic breakthroughs in the balance*. Available through: <https://freedomhouse.org/report/freedom-world/freedom-world-2013> [accessed 27 August 2015].

Gefenas, E., 2001. Is 'failure to thrive' syndrome relevant to Lithuanian healthcare ethics committees? *HEC Forum*, 13(4), pp. 381–92.

Hyder, A.A., Dawson, L., Bachani, A.M. and Lavery, J., 2009. Moving from research ethics review to research ethics systems in low-income and middle-income countries. *Lancet*, 373, pp. 862–5.

Jakusovaite, I. and Bankauskaite, V., 2007. Teaching ethics in a masters program in public health in Lithuania. *Journal of Medical Ethics*, 33, pp. 423–7.

Kovács, L., 2010. Implementation of clinical ethics consultation in conflict with professional conscience? Suggestions for reconciliation. In: J. Schildmann, J.S. Gordon and J. Vollmann eds., *Clinical ethics consultation: theories and methods, implementation, evaluation*. Farnham: Ashgate Publishing Ltd, pp. 65–78.

Kubar, O., 2010. *The current state of bioethics education in the system of medical education in the CIS member states*. Saint Petersburg: Publishing House of Saint Petersburg Pasteur Institute.

Lebeer, G., 2005. Clinical ethics committees in Europe: assistance in medical decisions, fora for democratic debates, or bodies to monitor basic rights? In: J. Gunning and S. Holm eds., *Ethics, law and society*, volume 1. Farnham: Ashgate Publishing Ltd, pp. 65–72.

Meulenbergs, T., Vermylen, J. and Schotsmans, P.T., 2005. The current state of clinical ethics and healthcare ethics committees in Belgium. *Journal of Medical Ethics*, 31(6), pp. 318–21.

Ministry of Health of the Republic of Belarus, 1999. *Model guidelines for healthcare ethics committees (in Russian). The Order No.131 on 22 April 1999*. Available through: <www.lawbelarus.com/repub2013/library156/legalact456296.htm> [accessed 31 August 2015].

Ministry of Health of the Republic of Belarus, 2006. *On establishment of the National Medical Ethics Committee (in Russian). The Order No.893 on 27 November 2006*. Available through: <www.lawbelarus.com/repub2013/library130/legalact430659. htm> [accessed 31 August 2015].

Ministry of Health of the Republic of Belarus, 2008. *Model guidelines for healthcare ethics committees (in Russian). The Order No.205 on 28 November 2008*. Available through: <minzdrav.gov.by/lcfiles/000127_178497_N205_2008.doc> [accessed 31 August 2015].

NRLRB: National Register of Legislation of the Republic of Belarus, 2008. *Law on the healthcare system of the Republic of Belarus (in Russian)*. Available through: <www.pravo.by/main.aspx?guid=3871&p0=v19302435&p2={NRPA}> [accessed 31 August 2015].

OSCE/ODIHR: Organization for Security and Co-operation in Europe Office for Democratic Institutions and Human Rights, 2010. *Belarus, presidential election, 19 December 2010. OSCE/ODIHR Election Observation Mission Report*. Warsaw, Organization for Security and Co-operation in Europe.

Richardson, E., Malakhova, I., Novik, I. and Famenka, A., 2013. Belarus: health system review. *Health Systems in Transition*, 15(5), pp. 1–118.

Sen, A., 1999. *Development as freedom*. New York: Anchor Books.

Siegler, M., Pellegrino, E.D. and Singer, P.A., 1990. Clinical medical ethics. *Journal of Clinical Ethics*, 1, pp. 5–9.

Silis, V., 2010. Research ethics system in Latvia: structure, functioning and problems. *Dilemata*, 2, pp. 55–69.

Steinkamp, N., Gordijn, B., Borovećki, A., Gefenas, E., Glasa, J., Guerrier, M. *et al.*, 2007. Regulation of healthcare committees in Europe. *Medicine, Health Care, and Philosophy*, 10(4), pp. 461–75.

Stüber, C., 2010. Ethics consultation: facilitating reflection on professional norms in medicine. In: J. Schildmann, J.S. Gordon and J. Vollmann eds., *Clinical ethics consultation: theories and methods, implementation, evaluation*. Farnham: Ashgate Publishing Ltd, pp. 79–88.

Swick, H.M., 1998. Academic medicine must deal with the clash of business and professional values. *Academic Medicine*, 73, pp. 751–5.

Swick, H.M., 2000. Toward a normative definition of medical professionalism. *Academic Medicine*, 75, pp. 612–16.

The World Bank, 2015. *Doing business 2015 going beyond efficiency. Economy Profile 2015 Belarus*. Washington, DC: The World Bank. [pdf.] Available through: <www. doingbusiness.org/reports/global-reports/~/media/giawb/doing%20business/ documents/profiles/country/BLR.pdf> [accessed 27 August 2015].

Tichtchenko, P. and Yudin, B., 1997. The moral status of fetuses in Russia. *Cambridge Quarterly of Healthcare Ethics*, 6(1), pp. 31–8.

Transparency International, 2014. *Corruption Perceptions Index: CPI 2014 Results*. Available through: <www.transparency.org/cpi2014/results> [accessed 27 August 2015].

UNDP: United Nations Development Programme Country Office in Belarus, 2005. *Belarus: addressing imbalances in the economy and society*. National Human Development Report 2004–2005. Available through: <www.by.undp.org/content/dam/belarus/ docs/NHDR_eng.pdf> [accessed 27 August 2015].

Vollmann, J., 2010. The implementation process of clinical ethics consultation: concepts, resistance, recommendations. In: J. Schildmann, J.S. Gordon and J. Vollmann eds., *Clinical ethics consultation: theories and methods, implementation, evaluation*. Farnham: Ashgate Publishing Ltd, pp. 91–108.

Wynia, M.K., Latham, S.R., Kao, A.C., Berg, J.W. and Emanuel, L.L., 1999. Medical professionalism in society. *New England Journal of Medicine*, 341, pp. 1612–16.

Yen, B.M. and Schneiderman, L.J., 1999. Impact of pediatric ethics consultations on patients, families, social workers, and physicians. *Journal of Perinatology*, 19, pp. 373–8.

8 Ethical problems concerning the international brain drain of healthcare professionals

Dorina Maria Stănescu

The problem

The 'brain drain' is not a new issue in philosophy and other disciplines.[1] This expression incorporates the migration of skilled workers from poor and developing countries to developed countries. Software developers, engineers, researchers in all fields and healthcare professionals (HPs) are leaving their countries of birth and education in search of opportunities to improve their lives. The brain drain is a special concern for the medical sector, because it results in large shortages in the number of HPs who stay in their country of birth and education (Docquier and Marfouk, 2006; Robinson and Clark, 2008; Eyal and Hurst, 2008; Haupt and Janeba, 2009). It seems that education cannot guarantee their staying in the country which needs them most, and educating more doctors in developing countries does not guarantee proper medical care for the citizens of that country in the long run (Groenhout, 2012).

The international brain drain problem first appeared in the 1940s when many Europeans emigrated to the USA and UK. By the end of 1979, the WHO reported that almost 90 per cent of migrating HPs went to Canada, Australia, the UK, the USA and Germany (Ahmad, 2004). The World Bank Report from October 2011 shows that there was a global shortage of 4.3 million HPs, which included doctors, nurses, midwives and support workers. A third of the global population lacks regular access to essential medicine (World Bank, 2011).

Nowadays, the phenomenon of the brain drain is still present, even though countries are trying to find solutions for it. The recent WHO assembly in 2013 tried to find ways to undermine the detrimental effects of the brain drain of HPs. They proposed that states adopt universal health coverage for all people, regardless of their status, so that poverty does not stand in the way of achieving health (WHO, 2013).

There are also inequalities between states regarding the number of existing HPs. According to the data available from WHO in 2009, the number of practising physicians in Romania was 48,484, with a density rate of 22.69 per 10,000 population, while the number of nurses and midwives was 125,699 with a density of 58.82 per 10,000 population (GHODR, Romania, 2014). By contrast, in 2010, Spain registered the number of nurses and midwives at 224,800 with a density of 51.1 per 10,000 population, and the number of physicians was 174,100 with a density of 39.57 per 10,000 population (GHODR, Spain, 2014). However, these figures are changing continuously.

Statistics from the OECD reveal that the number of physicians in developed countries is increasing. The number of practising physicians from Spanish hospitals, for example, increased from 135,800 in 2002 to 195,600 in 2011. The same situation can be encountered in the number of practising nurses in Spain, which grew from 168,833 in 2002 to 245,300 in 2012. Spain registered a total of 1,277,071 workers in healthcare and the social field in 2008 (OECD, 2013). The most promising figures are to be found in Sweden, where the density of midwives and nurses was 118.61 per 10,000 inhabitants in 2008, four times higher than in Romania (GHODR, Sweden, 2014). The density of practising physicians in 2009 was 3.8 per 1,000 inhabitants for Sweden and 3.54 per 1,000 inhabitants for Spain. Despite the visible increase in the number of medical personnel, hospitals and care centres are especially in need of nurses, and the continuously increasing numbers of old people will constantly point in this direction. As the number of patients increases, the need for healthcare also increases. We can predict, therefore, that, at least in an ageing Europe, there will be an extensive need for healthcare and, implicitly, for HPs.

The need for medical professionals encourages countries to attract and employ people from all over the world. Rich countries have more resources for undertaking these types of actions, and poor and developing countries are often the sources of emigration. Skilled doctors and nurses from poor and developing countries are most likely to respond to the call in the search for their own well-being (Katseli, Lucas and Xenogiani, 2006). Countries have to respond to these problems, because a small number of healthcare personnel cannot provide effective services in a system that is structurally and systemically fragile. If trained HPs migrate, countries will lose the resources invested in their education. If a country is left without skilled workers or specialists, then it will become unstable, politically, socially and economically. According to human rights, HPs are entitled to pursue their own well-being and right to free movement, and this is rational and reasonable. The problem is that the condition of people who live in poor and developing countries is worsening and someone has to take responsibility for it (Katseli *et al.*, 2006; WHO, 2013).

The problem is compounded when we subscribe responsibilities, duties or obligations to institutions or individuals without trying to justify our actions, so-called 'duty dumping'. An example may be to say that HPs have a duty or obligation to reside in their country of origin if it is affected by the brain drain. The important thing is that we cannot 'dump' responsibilities or obligations onto them, without solid justification and reasons. To infer that they have this duty only because HPs produce healthcare goods and, at the same time, are healthcare resources, is similar to saying that if they can do something, they ought to do it (Buchanan and Decamp, 2006, p. 97).

Some ethical concerns regarding healthcare professionals

On the other hand, there are several ethical concerns that HPs face or should think about when migrating. One of them is whether they should promote their own well-being and leave their country, causing a lack of human resources in the field of healthcare. We have to be aware that people from countries with poor resources would prefer to reside in their country of birth if they had a real choice that did not put them at a disadvantage. There is a need for stability and most people do not want to leave their country of origin, as Van Eyck shows by the example of a Polish nurse:

> Even though I see the many problems here (I also earn low wages), I try to look for other solutions instead of thinking about migrating. What influences this decision strongly is the family situation, family stability, the need to stay where I am living, the need to stay beside my family, my parents, my closest family. Really, if I have decent wages, and I have the possibility to support myself, if I have a house or an apartment, there's no need for me to migrate. I'm connected with this country, I'm closely connected with my family. However, if the situation is too difficult, I might have to leave.
>
> (Van Eyck, 2004, p. 17)

Another issue to be explored is whether HPs have a duty towards their co-nationals. This is a vast area of research and my intention here is only to indicate the two main points of view. Communitarians and nationalist scholars would say that since HPs are also citizens of their country of birth, they have a duty to their peers (Walzer, 1983; McIntyre, 1984; Taylor, 1989; Sandel, 2009; Bell and de-Shalit, 2011). The main argument is that since their birth, people residing in the same state begin to cooperate and to create duties between each other, duties that cannot just be given up so simply. Conversely, the cosmopolitan view tells us that citizens of each country should be allowed to move freely around the world and to reside anywhere they wish (Carens, 1992, 1995; Appiah, 2007; Abizadeh, 2008).

I embrace Robert Nozick's view in the sense that if we choose to cooperate, we owe others what the terms of a formal contract signed in total mutual agreement requires, and no other duties after the cooperation is finished (Nozick, 1974, p. 185). The fact that we are born in certain countries is arbitrary and we do not have the opportunity to agree to social cooperation from the start. In this sense, the doctors do not owe anything special to the people of the country in which they were born and educated.

Effects of the brain drain of healthcare professionals

Negative effects

The brain drain of HPs brings with it some effects not only for the people from the migrants' country of origin, but also for the population in the receiving countries.

First, we can observe the effect of the brain drain on the migrants' co-nationals, present and future generations, not only as individuals but as a community as well. Second, the effects are both negative and positive. There are people who do not like foreigners coming into their countries and who consider them intruders. However, this attitude does not extend to HPs, perhaps because everyone fears illness, pain or death, and doctors and nurses are 'tools' that can help to fight these fears. HPs receive positive discrimination perhaps because of their utility and importance for a person's well-being. A recent report from the European Commission considers HPs as very required on the job market (EC, 2014). Appealing to common sense, we can agree that there are people who dislike having outsiders in their country. They do not agree with having people near them who can cause harm in some way, are afraid for their security and well-being, have increased respect for the law, and so on. In the case of HPs, they are accepted not only because they are skilled workers who can improve the economic aspects of people's lives, but mostly because everyone needs medical care. The quality and quantity of health providers can make patients feel more secure that they are receiving good treatment.

Another negative effect of the brain drain is that the inequalities between individuals and states are increasing because of countries that are creating policies which foster only highly skilled workers. Therefore, a sort of structural injustice is taking place, as Lisa Eckenwiler observes:

> All in all, the migration of healthcare workers both reflects and perpetuates structural injustice. Structural injustice occurs where social and economic norms and processes serve systematically to undermine or constrain some people's abilities to develop their capacities, to determine their actions and the conditions of their actions, and threaten their equality, while at the same time enhancing and expanding others' prospects.
>
> (Eckenwiler, 2009, p. 176)

Structural injustice can also be seen when people are coerced by society and the economy to train in fields in which they do not actually want to work. Countries might need to train more and more health specialists, for example, because of the continuous need for healthcare and, thus, some people who would have liked to have had another career turn out to be doctors because they do not have any other job prospects. Perhaps a better organisation of the healthcare system could prevent this from happening.

Accepting only skilled workers from poor and developing countries could lead to the collapse of their economy and mean they will need more help from outside. They will be unable to progress without constant assistance. Additionally, a very troubling possibility is that poor and developing countries will be left without any trained and specialised professionals to teach future generations. I am optimistic we will find appropriate solutions before we reach this state of affairs, so that it will not happen.

Positive effects

There are also positive aspects regarding the migration of HPs, which are seen only if they return to the country of origin. If they do not return, but settle down in another country with their family, the patients and community that HPs leave behind will be disadvantaged. If they return, however, the patients and community can benefit from their knowledge: prospective HPs could learn how to improve in their work, and patients could receive better treatment. When it comes to the community of HPs from the receiving country, I believe they can benefit from having colleagues with other backgrounds. Both sides are likely to benefit if curing patients is the common ground. If an HP returns to their country of birth, the positive aspect for the patients in the country of origin is that the HP may have the opportunity to contribute to developing research and find better cures for illnesses due to the knowledge gained from working in more developed countries. It is very possible that research in poor and developing countries is less advanced because of a lack of funds, while funding in developed countries could cause the blooming of research.

There is also a push factor from developing and poor countries towards emigration. The return of migrants to their home countries could lead to a number of benefits, including the reversal of some of the adverse brain drain effects associated with the emigration of highly skilled workers, the transfer of knowledge and skills acquired by migrants abroad, and the creation of local businesses by migrants based on savings generated during employment abroad.

Moreover, migrants who intend to return – especially those with families in their home countries – can be expected to remit more of their wages than migrants who intend (and are permitted) to reside abroad on a permanent basis. There are positive aspects, such as a bigger income, remittances, high-tech training and better specialisation. There are doctors who return to the country of origin and try to apply what they learn, for example, by opening new private clinics.

Although the empirical evidence on this issue is mixed, there is some evidence that remittances initially increase, but eventually decrease with a migrant's duration of stay in the host country. This reflects the counteracting forces of wage increases (which increase remittances), on the one hand, and, on the other hand, increased detachment from the home country and family reunification (lowering remittances) over time (Carling, 2008; Ruhs, 2008).

Possible solutions

John Connell argued in *Migration and the Globalisation of Health Care: The Health Worker Exodus* (2010) that the main factor influencing migration is a major inequality in the economic sector and social development at a global level. It is very important to have adequate financial support to ensure the appropriate wages and working conditions in the healthcare system, since economic and social development influence the retention of health workers (Connell, 2010, p. 94).

There are several possible solutions to avoid the brain drain of healthcare personnel. One option could be changing or reforming the education system to institute a formal contract between the state and the taxpayers regarding the citizens' desire for healthcare. How much of their income, for example, should be transferred to healthcare and how much to other domains. If they want to pay two per cent of their income to healthcare and four per cent to education, the government should allow them to do that rather than coercing them into paying a strict percentage. According to this view, people are entitled to the results of whatever they pay for in terms of taxes. For the time being, however, this idea is very utopian, at least for some states such as Romania, where the government allocates the money from public taxes without having in mind a citizen's will in respect of their particular needs or desires.

Alternatively, the contract could be between the state and the future doctors. At the end of a doctor's training, if this was paid by the public sector, they must stay in the country to work in the healthcare system. This kind of contract is also made in the private sector between the employer and the employee where there is a contract regarding training.

Both these solutions could engender positive effects, but, of course, they have to be tested in order to find out the most suitable path towards reducing the brain drain of HPs.

When there are not enough doctors or nurses in the public system, those with sufficient personal resources are able to go to private hospitals or clinics. Another option is to accede to medical tourism: to be a global patient who can move to different places and be attended by qualified personnel around the world. Again, this is only possible for those who have sufficient resources to be able to go to high-quality clinics or hospitals in any country they desire and in which they can find the highly trained HPs they need.

There is also the argument that open borders make private investments in education more attractive. Poutvaara and Kanniainen (2000) try to prove in their analysis that the gain from the positive incentive effect can dominate the negative effect from the brain drain and, thus, increase human capital in the home country. Another possible solution is a redistributive tax scheme to be used for educational subsidies. This could help communities support the creation of new medical personnel or other skilled workers. Poutvaara and Kanniainen show that social contracts of financing higher education on a national level break down when skilled workers emigrate. However, even if social contracts might break down, reinforcing the agreements by other types of contracts which provide sufficient information to the parties and also the possibility to choose might be a solution (Poutvaara and Kanniainen, 2000).

People who pay for their education should be allowed to do whatever they want with the skills that they have acquired, provided that their use is morally and legally legitimate. Taking Locke's idea that when a person mixes their labour with some previously unowned object, the latter becomes their possession, then it could be argued that HPs are entitled to the skills they have acquired (Laslett, 1960, II, sect.27). The doctors have earned their freedom through work. If individuals pay for their training and education, then there is no obligation of repayment on their behalf. A doctor educated in Romania can be said to have a duty to compensate for the education received, but not for becoming a doctor. In order to become a doctor, more than education in the medical field is needed. A lot of personal effort and talent, many hours of work and possibly personal sacrifices must be made. Therefore, in addition to education, which is a key aspect, a lot of personal effort and work is required in order to become a doctor. This is the same for all other occupations. If education is something previously unowned and the effort one allocates to becoming a doctor is considered work, mixing those two elements may lead to fair appropriation and ownership of resources. In this case, being a doctor is transformed into a personal merit, even if public education or the help of others contributed to this status. Under this framework, medical personnel have the liberty to use their work however they see fit or appropriate, and they have the liberty to migrate to any country they want.

One way the problem could be fixed is by changing the institutional framework. Denying the access of any individual, skilled or unskilled, to free movement and ownership of their own body, work and skills is very unjust if we respect the principles of a free society. It is our duty to find pull factors which could be incorporated into policies and could somehow create incentives and opportunities for skilled workers to stay in their own country. However, there should be no restriction from outside or any regulation regarding free movement and the use of their skills.

Countries could call into question assumptions about shortages and also think about ways to promote policies that foster health. There is also the possibility of training more healthcare workers and introducing a temporary migration scheme, so that they are coerced to return to the donor country (Record and Mohiddin, 2006).

Conclusion

There are several ethical concerns regarding the international brain drain of HPs. There is a need for more awareness regarding these aspects both in the medical profession and in public life in general. There are some solutions to the brain drain of HPs, but there are still many questions without suitable answers which can be incorporated into the current political framework. As beneficial as the continuing debate between scholars and policy-makers might be, the ideal solution is hard to achieve. More research is needed at the domestic level as well as internationally.

Note

1 The ideas presented here are also in some parts of my doctoral thesis: *A Moral Investigation of the Brain Drain of Healthcare Professionals: The Rawls-Nozick Debate Framework*, 2014 (unpublished).

References

Abizadeh, A., 2008. Democratic theory and border coercion. No right to unilaterally control your own borders. *Political Theory*, 36, pp. 37–65.

Ahmad, O.B., 2004. Brain drain: the flight of human capital. *Bulletin of the World Health Organization*, 82, pp. 797–8.

Appiah, K.A., 2007. *Cosmopolitanism: ethics in a world of strangers*. New York: Norton.

Bell, D. and de-Shalit, A., 2011. *The spirit of cities: why the identity of a city matters in a global age*. Princeton, NJ: Princeton University Press.

Buchanan, A. and Decamp, M., 2006. Responsibility for global health. *Theoretical Medicine and Bioethics*, 27, pp. 95–114.

Carens, J., 1992. Migration and morality: a liberal egalitarian perspective. In: B. Barry and R.E. Goodin eds., *Free movement: ethical issues in the transnational migration of people and of money*. University Park, PA: Pennsylvania State University Press, pp. 25–47.

Carens, J., 1995. Aliens and citizens: the case for open borders. In: R. Beiner ed., *Theorizing citizenship*. Albany, NY: State University of New York Press, pp. 229–53.

Carling, J., 2008. The determinants of migrant remittances. *Oxford Review of Economic Policy*, 24(3), pp. 582–99.

Connell, J., 2010. *Migration and the globalisation of health care: the health worker exodus*. London: Edward Elgar Publishing Limited.

Docquier, F. and Marfouk, A., 2006. International migration by education attainment, (1990–2000). In: C. Özden and M. Schiff eds., *International migration, remittances and the brain drain*. Washington, DC: The World Bank and Palgrave Macmillan, ch. 5.

EC: European Commission, 2014. Mapping and analysing bottleneck vacancies in EU labour markets. [online] Available through: <http://ec.europa.eu/social/main.jsp?langId=en&catId=89&newsId=2131&furtherNews=yes> [accessed 28 August 2015].

Eckenwiler, L.A., 2009. Care worker migration and transnational justice. *Public Health Ethics*, 2(2), pp. 171–83.

Eyal, N. and Hurst, S.A., 2008. Physician brain drain: can nothing be done? *Public Health Ethics*, 1(2), pp. 180–92.

GHODR: Global Health Observatory Data Repository, Romania, 2014. [online] Available through: <http://apps.who.int/gho/data/node.country.country-ROU?lang=en> [accessed 14 April 2015].

GHODR: Global Health Observatory Data Repository, Spain, 2014. [online] Available through: <http://apps.who.int/gho/data/node.country.country-ESP?lang=en> [accessed 14 April 2015].

GHODR: Global Health Observatory Data Repository, Sweden, 2014. [online] Available through: <http://apps.who.int/gho/data/node.country.country-SWE?lang=en> [accessed 14 April 2015].

Groenhout, R., 2012. The 'brain drain' problem: migrating medical professionals and global health care. *International Journal of Feminist Approaches to Bioethics*, 5(1), pp. 1–24.

Haupt, A. and Janeba, E., 2009. Education, redistribution and the threat of brain drain. *International Tax and Public Finance*, 16, pp. 1–24.

Katseli, L.T., Lucas, R.E.B. and Xenogiani, T., 2006. *Effect of migration on sending countries: what do we know?* OECD Development Centre, Working Paper, 250. [pdf] Available through: <www.un.org/esa/population/migration/turin/Symposium_ Turin_files/P11_Katseli> [accessed 24 June 2015].

Laslett, P., ed., 1960. *Two treatises of government. John Locke.* Cambridge: Cambridge.

McIntyre, A., 1984. *After virtue.* 2nd ed. Notre-Dame, IN: University of Notre Dame Press.

Nozick, R., 1974. *Anarchy, state and utopia.* New York: Basic Books.

OECD: Organisation for Economic Co-operation and Development, 2013. *Statistics on health.* [online] Available through: <http://stats.oecd.org/index.aspx?DataSet Code=HEALTH_STAT> [accessed 21 June 2015].

OECD: Organisation for Economic Co-operation and Development, 2014. *International migration outlook 2014.* Paris: OECD Publishing. [online] Available through: <http:// dx.doi.org/10.1787/migr_outlook-2014-en> [accessed 21 June 2015].

Poutvaara, P. and Kanniainen, V., 2000. Why invest in your neighbor? Social contract on educational investment. *International Tax and Public Finance*, 7(4), pp. 547–62.

Record, R. and Mohiddin, A., 2006. An economic perspective on Malawi's medical 'brain drain'. *Globalization and Global Health*, 2(1), pp. 1–8.

Robinson, M. and Clark, P., 2008. Forging solutions to health worker migration. *The Lancet*, 371, pp. 391–2.

Ruhs, M., 2008. Economic research and labour immigration policy. *Oxford Review of Economic Policy*, 24(3), pp. 403–26.

Sandel, M., 2009. *Justice – what's the right thing to do?* New York: Farrar, Straus and Giroux.

Taylor, C., 1989. *Sources of the self: the making of modern identity.* Cambridge, MA: Harvard University Press.

Van Eyck, K., 2004. *Women and international migration in the health sector.* France: Ferney-Voltaire PSI.

Walzer, M., 1983. *Spheres of justice.* New York: Basic Books.

WHO: World Health Organisation, 2013. *Research for universal health coverage.* Word Health Report 2013. [online] Available through: <www.who.int/whr/2013/ report/en/index.html> [accessed 2 September 2015].

World Bank, 2011. Report October 2011. [online] Available through: <http://web. worldbank.org/WBSITE/EXTERNAL/EXTABOUTUS/EXTANNREP/ EXTANNREP2011/0,,menuPK:8070643~pagePK:64168427~piPK:64168435~ theSitePK:8070617,00.html> [accessed 2 September 2015].

Part IV

Professional leadership and team decision-making in healthcare

9 Substituted or supported decisions?

Examining models of decision-making within interprofessional team decision-making for individuals at risk of lacking decision-making capacity

*Gemma Clarke, Sarah Galbraith,
Jeremy Woodward, Anthony Holland
and Stephen Barclay*

Background

Interprofessional decision-making and artificial nutrition

Interprofessional teams are used increasingly in healthcare to make difficult ethical decisions (D'Amour *et al.*, 2005; Légaré *et al.*, 2011; Weinberger *et al.*, 2015). However, there is only limited literature on how interprofessional teams make difficult decisions regarding patients with multiple comorbidities and complex illnesses (Clarke *et al.*, 2013; Weinberger *et al.*, 2015). Two such complex decisions concern artificial nutrition and hydration for individuals with neurological conditions who may have some degree of cognitive impairment.

Artificial nutrition is more than just assistance with eating and drinking. Artificial nutrition can be delivered directly into the gut, which is known as enteral feeding (NCCAC, 2006), or intravenously, referred to as parenteral feeding (Singer *et al.*, 2009). Common methods of enteral feeding are nasogastric (NG), in which a narrow plastic tube is passed through the nose into the stomach, and percutaneous endoscopic gastrostomy (PEG), in which a tube is inserted directly into the stomach through the abdominal wall under local anaesthetic. Hydration by artificial means can also be given intravenously or subcutaneously (GMC, 2010).

Many people with neurological conditions may find that they are unable to eat and drink as usual, particularly as their condition continues or worsens. People, for example, with dementia (Mitchell *et al.*, 2009), intellectual and physical disabilities, such as motor neurone disease (Gravestock, 2000) and acquired brain injuries (Corrigan *et al.*, 2011; Mackay, Morgan and Bernstein, 2013) can find they are unable to take food and fluids orally and/or might require additional support during mealtimes. When this occurs, decisions concerning artificial methods of nutrition and hydration could be required.

Difficult ethical decision-making

Decisions about artificial nutrition and hydration are often challenging. They might involve issues of life and death: weighing the potential for increased morbidity and prolonged suffering with the potential of a shortened life if no intervention takes place. Competing human rights have to be measured and balanced, such as the right to life (European Convention on Human Rights, Article 2; ECHR, 1950) and the right to freedom from degrading treatment (Article 3; ECHR, 1950). The lack of a strong evidence base, particularly the dearth of randomised control trials, contributes to the difficulties because of uncertainty about clinical outcomes (RCP, 2010). Treatment decisions can be particularly challenging for some interventions, such as PEG. Percutaneous endoscopic gastrostomy insertions have been associated with futile procedures (Johnston, Tham and Mason, 2008), significant mortality and morbidity rates (Johnston *et al.*, 2008) and a lack of evidence of benefit in certain patient groups, such as those with advanced dementia (Candy, Sampson and Jones, 2009). These decisions are particularly difficult when someone is approaching the end of life, or when the individual in question lacks the mental capacity to be involved in the decision-making themselves. As with all medical treatments or interventions, valid informed consent of the patient is generally central, but many patients who might benefit from artificial nutrition and hydration could have illnesses that result in the person being unable to make an informed decision and these patients may have been judged as lacking the decision-making capacity to consent to the procedure (Clarke *et al.*, 2014).

Decisions for those at risk of lacking decision-making capacity

The United Nations Convention on the Rights of Persons with Disabilities (UNCRPD) requires signatory parties to protect and promote the full human rights of persons with disabilities, including those at risk of lacking decision-making capacity (UN, 2006). The UNCRPD views disability through the lens of human rights; Article 12 guarantees that persons with disabilities, 'enjoy legal capacity on an equal basis with others in all aspects of life' (UNCRPD, Article 12(2); UN, 2006). This means that countries must 'provide access by persons with disabilities to the support they may require in exercising their legal capacity' (UNCRPD, Article 12(3); UN, 2006). The move towards supported decision-making has been seen as a paradigm shift in human rights for people with disabilities (Dinerstein, 2012).

This model of supported decision-making aims to replace older models of traditional adult guardianship legislation which formally appoint a person, often a close family member, to act as a substitute decision-maker (Carney, 2014). Guardianship legislation has been criticised for its paternalism and denial of rights of people with impaired capacity (Carney, 2014). Conversely, supported decision-making is a series of practices, relationships and agreements of varying legal formality designed to assist an individual with a cognitive or physical disability to make decisions and communicate their choice (Dinerstein, 2012). Supported decision-making is not clearly defined within the UNCRDP and may refer to a wide range of differing practices. Important conceptual differences include distinctions between 'support with' decisions and 'supported decision-making', the connection to legal mental capacity, and differences in formal legal rulings and civil society schemes (Browning, Bigby and Douglas, 2014).

The Mental Capacity Act (MCA) 2005 (DH, 2007) provides a statutory framework within one jurisdiction, England and Wales, for how to proceed when people are judged not to have the mental capacity to make a particular decision. The Act states that a person is only considered to be lacking decision-making capacity for a particular decision if all of the following criteria apply: the person has a disorder or impairment of the brain or mind, all practical steps have been taken without success, and they are unable to understand the relevant information, retain the information, weigh the information and communicate their decision. Within Scotland, decision-making is covered by the Adults With Incapacity (Scotland) Act (2000). Similarly, in most US jurisdictions, individuals are expected to be able to demonstrate four abilities to show decision-making capacity: appreciate the nature and consequences of their own situation, understand the relevant information, be able to reason about potential risks and benefits, and communicate a choice (Sessums, Zembrzuska and Jackson, 2011).

The MCA 2005 requires that any decision made for an individual lacking the capacity to make a specific decision is in accordance with their 'best interests'. Best interests are defined broadly, including not making assumptions on the basis of age, appearance, condition or behaviour (DH, 2007), but also importantly, the person requiring the decision to be made must consider the individual's past views and the views of family and others close to the person in question. Advance decisions to refuse treatment must be followed if valid and applicable, even if it might result in the person's death (DH, 2009). Expressions of treatment preferences or 'advance expressions of preferences' are not legally binding, but should be incorporated as part of the decision-making process when assessing 'best interests' (DH, 2009).

Substituted versus supported decision-making

Some critics have argued that assessments of capacity within the MCA 2005 might not be compliant with the UNCRPD (Dhanda, 2007; Salzman, 2010). A strong reading of Article 12 of the UNCRPD rejects the very concept of decision-making incompetence, arguing that there is no point at which legal capacity should be considered to be lost (Dhanda, 2007). Such approaches push the focus away from capacity testing and substituted decision-making towards an evaluative approach to decision-making abilities in which a person's support requirements for decision-making are determined and then met (Gooding, 2013).

This study examines differing models of supported and substituted decision-making within interprofessional team ethical decisions. It utilises a thematic analysis (Braun and Clarke, 2006) and draws upon the findings from a previous study examining decision-making in a UK hospital-based interprofessional team concerning patients with complex feeding difficulties (Clarke *et al.*, 2015).

Methods

Setting

The setting for this research was the UK hospital Feeding Issues Multi-Professional Team (FIMPT), which meets weekly to discuss patients with complex feeding difficulties and aims to improve decision-making concerning assessment, treatment and clinical outcomes. The team comprises medical members from the departments of Gastroenterology, Palliative Care, Medicine for the Elderly, Speech and Language Therapy, Dietetics, Nutrition Clinical Nurse Specialists and Endoscopy nurses. The team meets for around one hour weekly to discuss patients who have been referred. The FIMPT meetings are part of normal clinical practice; they are not held as 'best interests' proceedings. For further background on the setting, see Clarke *et al.* (2015).

Data collection and analysis

A thematic analysis approach was utilised for fieldwork, data analysis and inter-pretation (Braun and Clarke, 2006). Detailed field notes on open topics were taken for the first two months. For the last month, a subset of four meetings was sampled. These meetings were audio-recorded and analysed alongside the detailed field notes. Notes were anonymised and the audio recordings were transcribed and anonymised. All notes and transcriptions were entered into NVivo 9 (QSR International) for analysis.

A six-stage process was undertaken for the thematic analysis: (1) Familiarisation with the data. The first author relistened to the audio recordings and read and reread the transcripts. (2) Initial coding stage. The transcripts were coded using both open inductive data-driven coding and then coded using three broad categories derived from the research questions. (3) Searching for themes. The initial codes were discussed in team meetings between authors GC, SB and AH. Insights from theory were discussed and initial descriptive codes were developed into higher level analytical themes. (4) Reviewing the themes. The themes were reviewed and refined in an on-going process of working with data in NVivo and discussing the findings in team meetings. (5) Defining and naming the themes. The themes were refined and reviewed by discussion. These were broadly separated into two overarching themes: the decision-making process model and the interdependent decision-making axes, with six and four sub-themes, respectively. (6) Producing the report. The final themes were written up to produce the paper which was reviewed and edited by all authors.

The retrospective analysis of records was undertaken using an electronic search of the hospital's computer system for all FIMPT reports in 2011. Data was extracted into an anonymised form. Descriptive statistical analysis was undertaken using PASW Statistics 17 (IBM Corp).

Ethics

After a review of the evaluation protocol by the committee Chair of the National Health Service (NHS) Research Ethics Committee Cambridgeshire 2, it was agreed on 3 August 2011 that the project was classed as a service evaluation and would not require further review by the committee. The researcher undertaking the fieldwork was awarded an honorary contract with the NHS Trust to undertake this work: this bound the researcher to the same standards of conduct and confidentiality as paid employees of the NHS Trust. This evaluation was carried out in compliance with the World Medical Association Declaration of Helsinki (WMA, 1964).

Anonymity, access and informed consent

The gender of all patients mentioned in this article has been redacted and the year in which the study was undertaken has been removed to protect anonymity. Quotations have been edited to redact gender.

After a review of the evaluation protocol, verbal consent was taken from the core members of the FIMPT team. Written informed consent for the quotations used was taken from the key team members.

Results

Patient characteristics

During the one-month sample of audio-recorded meetings, 12 patients were referred and 17 separate discussions were held. The largest group to be referred were those with a primary diagnosis of cancer (five individuals, 42 per cent of all those referred). The remaining seven patients referred had primary diagnoses of cerebrovascular accident, motor neurone disease, Parkinson's disease, heart disease, pneumonia, Down's syndrome with dementia and dementia. Of this subset of 12 patients, half (50 per cent) had decision-making capacity throughout the entire decision-making process. Five patients (42 per cent) had no or unclear decision-making capacity at one point in the decision-making process or had no/unclear capacity during the entire decision-making process. For one patient (8 per cent), no statement was made about their decision-making capacity.

All patient cases, both with and without decision-making capacity, were analysed. The analysis focused upon only those cases involving patients with no or unclear decision-making capacity for the analysis of factors involved in making decisions and the examination of the different models of decision-making.

Balancing complex and multifaceted decision-making factors

Decisions concerning artificial nutrition and hydration for patients at risk of lacking decision-making capacity were complex and multifaceted. The topics of discussion varied for each individual case, but the outcome of decision-making relied upon weighting and balancing the information available along four different but interdependent axes. A model of these axes has been created including: (1) risks, burdens and benefits; (2) treatment goals; (3) normative ethical values; and (4) interested parties (see Table 9.1). These axes of decision-making are completely interdependent. All available information for each decision has to be weighted or considered in relation to each axis, which, in turn, has to be considered and reconsidered in relation to the other axes.

For further discussion of the decision-making axes, see Clarke *et al.* (2015).

The decision-making process

The process of decision-making observed at each interprofessional meeting followed a similar format. A model has been created to describe this process consisting of the following parts: (1) forming the picture; (2) identifying the problem; (3) discussion; and (4) outcome and planning. The meeting is led by the Chair, who is usually the Consultant in Palliative Care (see Table 9.2). In the first stage, *forming the picture*, the patient's case is presented by a member of the clinical team who knows the patient, and then the dietician and the speech and language therapist present the results from their assessments. In stage two, *identifying the problem*, the Chair and other participants will ask further questions across the multi-professional team attending the meeting.

Table 9.1 Model of decision-making axes upon which clinical information was weighted to make decisions

Decision-making axes	Description
Risks, burdens and benefits	Comparison and weighting of the different treatment options and interventions by their potential effectiveness, dangers, outcomes and side-effects.
Treatment goals	The intended outcome specific to a particular treatment/intervention, place (institution/home) for future care for the patient or the overall intended outcome.
Normative ethical values	A balancing of actions in terms of ethical value. Actions in terms of their utilitarian value, i.e. increasing patient well-being and/or longevity, and deontological value, i.e. a 'good' course of action regardless of outcome.
Interested parties	Discussions incorporated the views of all stakeholders involved, which could include the patient or their previous wishes, clinical team, relatives, etc.

Table 9.2 Model of the process of FIMPT decision-making based on a three-month non-participant observation

Decision stage	Observation	Description
0. Before the meeting	Not observed	Patient referred from ward or community. The dietician, speech and language therapist, gastroenterologist and other relevant specialists assess the patient depending upon time of admission and time of referral. Decision-making capacity is assessed. Treatment options are talked over and explained with the patient and/or next of kin.
1. Forming the picture	Observed	Background information about the patient's case is presented by a member of the clinical team who knows the patient. Dietitian and speech and language therapist present the results of their assessments.
2. Identifying the problem	Observed	If the reasons for the patient's referral are apparent and their diagnosis is clear, the discussion can move straight onto stage three. In complex cases, the Chair and other participants will ask further questions of the person presenting the case, the speech and language therapist, dietician and anyone else who has examined the patient.
3. Discussion	Observed	A deeper conversation about potential treatments and interventions. Conversation seeks to balance risks and benefits, other clinical issues, and includes ethical and social concerns. At this stage, the discussion has a less structured format. Stage three continues until the weight of evidence for a particular treatment option or course of action becomes apparent.
4. Outcome and planning	Observed	The Chair states the outcome of the decision-making process and a brief discussion of treatment scheduling and planning follows. The outcome for some patients might involve further direct patient assessment by one of the FIMPT clinicians; or, it could involve referral to the Palliative Care or Medicine for the Elderly teams, who will assist in the future clinical management of the patient alongside nutrition management.
5. After the meeting	Not observed	The recommendations from the meeting are presented back to the patient and/or next of kin by the team handling the treatment who have presented the patient at the meeting. Further discussions and decision-making take place. Relevant scheduling and planning take place. The team handling the treatment return to the next meeting for further discussion if additional questions arise or if the patient's condition changes.

In stage three, *discussion*, the decision-making moves into a more in-depth conversation about potential treatments and interventions. The different professions discuss the risks and benefits, other clinical issues, and include ethical and social concerns. At this stage, the discussion has a less structured format. Stage three continues until the weight of evidence for a particular treatment option or course of action becomes apparent. In the last stage of the meeting, *outcome and planning*, the Chair states the outcome of the decision-making process and a brief discussion of treatment scheduling and planning follows. The outcome for some patients may involve further direct patient assessment by one of the FIMPT clinicians; or, it could involve referral to the Palliative Care or Medicine for the Elderly teams, who will assist in the future clinical management of the patient alongside nutrition management.

Decision-making was not a singular decision about one method of artificial nutrition, but rather a process of problem-solving for patients who often had complex symptomatology and multiple comorbidities. Decision-making was not limited to team meetings: patients were assessed on the ward before and after presentation at the FIMPT meeting, including an assessment of decision-making capacity. Discussions were on-going, taking place both before and after the meetings. These discussions involved the ward team, relatives and, if possible, the patient themselves. This included review by FIMPT Consultants, which might be required to assess the technical aspects of tube placement, issues regarding decision-making capacity, discussions regarding patient place of care for outpatients, and on-going specialist palliative care input providing symptom control and advance care planning. Multiple treatment options and interventions were considered for each individual patient, ranging from continued observation, through changes in medication regimens to interventions, such as PEG insertion.

Examples of substituted and supported decisions

Additional support could be provided for some patients with cognitive impairments to help them make decisions about the different methods of artificial nutrition:

> 'Yesterday when s/he said, "Oh not at the minute, can I think about it?" that's not normally her/him; if something's "No", it's a big "No", and it's quite loud . . . and s/he wasn't kind of as destructive as s/he was when we said about an NG tube. So I don't really know, I said to her/him I'd give her/him time. S/he said "Can I think about it?" So I said I'd give her/him some time and perhaps take the written information so s/he can . . . her/him and her/his mum can have a look through. And I said I'd take a tube up, so s/he could see what it would look like and how it would work and things like that, so s/he's fully aware of everything.'
>
> (Discussion of a patient with a primary diagnosis of cancer and learning/intellectual disability of unknown cause)

Though this patient was able to make the decision themselves with the support of their family and the interprofessional team, it is embedded within the context of the multistage FIMPT process (see Table 9.2 above). Discussions will have taken place before and after the meetings, and decisions, such as the referral to the FIMPT in the first place, might have been taken with or without involving the patient.

Some patients had a greater amount of cognitive and physical impairment. They lacked the capacity to participate in discussions about their health-care and the ability to communicate a choice about their care. However, a judgement by family members concerning what they would have wanted could be included in the decision–making process:

CLINICIAN 1: So we haven't got any reports of what family might think s/he would want in this situation or . . .

CLINICIAN 2: No.

CLINICIAN 1: . . . or what they support? This is probably quite important to establish before approaching with another NG.

(Discussion about an elderly patient with dementia and dysphagia)

In other cases, the patient lacked capacity to participate in a discussion about their healthcare and the ability to communicate a choice, and might never have had the capacity to make such decisions: for example, a patient who now spends most of their time asleep.

'S/he's uncommunicative and spends most of the day asleep or very, very drowsy, um, except . . . With the exception of if her/his family turn up, they will generally sort of . . . S/he'll perk up a little bit, open her/his eyes and kind of make some sounds but s/he's not really communicative.'

(Discussion of a patient with dementia and Down's syndrome)

In these cases, no support could be offered which could help the patient make and communicate their decision. However, as decisions were made in the patients' best interests, factors which appeared to make them happy, such as, in this case, the presence of their family, was incorporated into the decision–making.

Discussion

Interprofessional decision–making concerning feeding interventions for individuals who lack capacity is a dynamic and complex process. The decision–making in the FIMPT was not a one–off choice, but rather involved many different steps and many decisions. Discussions involving relatives and other clinicians were also part of the process, taking place both before and after team meetings. The decision–making process evolved as the patient's condition changed, sometimes involving re–referring and re–discussion at FIMPT meetings.

The study revealed a complex and often 'messy' reality of decision-making in the real world; decisions were always on-going, involving multiple recommendations and decision-makers. The study findings reveal there is no clear distinction between supported and substituted decision-making, because decisions in real-world clinical practice do not exist in isolation. Decisions involved multiple stages: some involved substituted decisions, such as deciding which treatments to recommend, others involved supported decision-making, such as taking into account a patient's behaviour even if they did not have full decision-making capacity.

The distinction between substituted and supported decision-making might be better conceptualised as a sliding scale in which parts of decisions requiring substitution decisions should always be in a patient's 'best interests', with capacity also being maximised for supporting decisions at the same time. The findings also reveal the importance and robustness of interprofessional discussions in these settings: the same level of debate could not be achieved by a uni-professional discussion. This chapter reports on a small-scale service evaluation: further research could helpfully compare these models of decision-making in both uni-professional and interprofessional teams.

Conclusions

Decisions surrounding stopping oral feeding and inserting feeding tubes are serious and challenging. The decision to intervene or not intervene with feeding often occurs under grave circumstances where continued life itself could be at stake. In this example of one hospital within the jurisdiction of England and Wales, interprofessional team meetings addressed these decisions using a formalised process operating within the framework of the MCA (DH, 2007), which requires decision-makers to act according to the patient's best interests. The perspectives of different disciplines concerning what might be the most appropriate course of action were encouraged and sought during discussions. The MCA also requires that the past and present views of the person concerned and their family are considered.

Decision-making regarding feeding interventions involves multiple decision-makers and decision points: it is acknowledged that the study has not addressed all of these, nor seen the entire picture. The ward Consultant responsible for the patient's care was not usually present at the meeting; the case often being presented by a junior member of the medical team. The study did not address how decision-making capacity had been assessed by the ward team, how it was reviewed by the FIMPT, or how information was relayed to patients and their families. The Consultant who would potentially insert the PEG was present for decisions concerning its insertion. However, the study did not include subsequent consultations with the patient and family after the team meeting to explain the decision to proceed with an intervention and obtain informed consent or assent. The multiple points of decision-making, and the number of people involved with the decision-making process mean there is a potential for anonymity of multiple decision-makers to arise. While the meetings operate within the MCA, what the present chapter describes does not constitute a 'best interests proceeding' under the MCA; instead it is part of routine clinical practice. The team did not assess decision-making capacity at meetings, but did review the assessments. The patients' relatives did not attend the meetings, but their views were sought. The team were one-step removed from the patient's bedside and, thus, unable to make 'best interests' decisions. It could be reasoned that the team meetings made healthcare or 'medical best interest' decisions, deciding on the right medical treatment while using MCA 'best interests' language.

Some legal interpretations argue that, under the UNCRPD, there is no point at which legal decision-making capacity is lost and, thus, all decisions must be supported rather than substituted (Dhanda, 2007; Salzman, 2010; Gooding, 2013). Legal capacity testing within the MCA in England and Wales represents a 'cut-off point' for a decision and creates a categorical distinction between supported and substituted decision-making. This study has illustrated that decisions in real-world interprofessional clinical practice may contain elements of both substituted and supported decision-making, often moving backwards and forwards between the two. Substituted and supported decision-making might be better represented as existing on a continuum.

Acknowledgements

This chapter presents independent research funded by the National Institute for Health Research Collaboration for Leadership in Applied Health Research and Care for Cambridgeshire and Peterborough at Cambridgeshire and Peterborough NHS Foundation Trust. The views expressed are those of the authors and not necessarily those of the NHS, the National Institute for Health Research or the Department of Health.

Competing interests

Authors SG and JW are members of the multi-professional team observed in this study. While they have had input into the writing of this chapter, the final decision as to the content rested with GC, SB and AH.

Author contributions

GC, AH and SB conceived and designed the research. GC undertook the fieldwork. GC, AH and SB analysed the data. GC, SG, JW, AH and SB wrote the chapter. All authors read and approved the final manuscript.

References

Braun, V. and Clarke, V., 2006. Using thematic analysis in psychology. *Qualitative Research in Psychology*, 3, pp. 77–101.

Browning, M., Bigby, C. and Douglas, J., 2014. Supported decision making: understanding how its conceptual link to legal capacity is influencing the development of practice. *Research and Practice in Intellectual and Developmental Disabilities*, 1, pp. 34–45.

Candy, B., Sampson, E. and Jones, L., 2009. Enteral tube feeding in older people with advanced dementia: findings from a Cochrane systematic review. *International Journal of Palliative Nursing*, 15, pp. 396–404.

Carney, T., 2014. Clarifying, operationalising, and evaluating supported decision making models. *Research and Practice in Intellectual and Developmental Disabilities*, 1, pp. 46–50.

Clarke, G., Galbraith, S., Woodward, J., Holland, A. and Barclay, S., 2014. Should they have a percutaneous endoscopic gastrostomy? The importance of assessing decision-making capacity and the central role of a multidisciplinary team. *Clinical Medicine*, 14, pp. 245–9.

Clarke, G., Galbraith, S., Woodward, J., Holland, A. and Barclay, S., 2015. Eating and drinking interventions for people at risk of lacking decision-making capacity: who decides and how? *BMC Medical Ethics*, 16:41.

Clarke, G., Harrison, K., Holland, A., Kuhn, I. and Barclay, S., 2013. How are treatment decisions made about artificial nutrition for individuals at risk of lacking capacity? A systematic literature review. *PLoS One*, 8, p. e61475.

Corrigan, M., Escuro, A., Celestin, J. and Kirby, D., 2011. Nutrition in the stroke patient. *Nutrition in Clinical Practice*, 26, pp. 242–52.

D'Amour, D., Ferrada-Videl, M., San Martin Rodriguez, L. and Beaulieu, M., 2005. The conceptual basis for interprofessional collaboration: core concepts and theoretical frameworks. *Journal of Interprofessional Care*, 19, pp. 116–31.

DH: Department of Health, 2007. *Mental Capacity Act 2005: Code of Practice*. London, Department of Health. Available through: <www.gov.uk/government/uploads/system/uploads/attachment_data/file/224660/Mental_Capacity_Act_code_of_practice.pdf> [accessed 11 September 2015].

DH: Department of Health, 2009. *Reference guide to consent for examination or treatment*, 2nd ed., London, Department of Health. Available through: <www.gov.uk/government/uploads/system/uploads/attachment_data/file/138296/dh_103653_1_.pdf> [accessed 11 September 2015].

Dhanda, A., 2007. Legal capacity in the disability rights convention: stranglehold of the past or lodestar for the future? *Syracuse Journal of International Law and Commerce*, 34, pp. 460–2.

Dinerstein, R., 2012. Implementing legal capacity under Article 12 of the UN Convention on the Rights of Persons with Disabilities: the difficult road from guardianship to supported decision-making. *Human Rights Brief*, 19, pp. 1–5.

ECHR: European Convention on Human Rights, 1950. European Court of Human Rights, Council of Europe. Available through: <www.echr.coe.int/Documents/Convention_ENG.pdf> [accessed 10 September 2015].

GMC: General Medical Council, 2010. *Treatment and care towards the end of life: good practice in decision making*. London: General Medical Council.

Gooding, P., 2013. Supported decision-making: a rights-based disability concept and its implications for mental health law. *Psychiatry, Psychology and Law*, 20, pp. 431–51.

Gravestock, S., 2000. Eating disorders in adults with intellectual disability. *Journal of Intellectual Disability Research*, 44, pp. 625–37.

Johnston, S., Tham, T. and Mason, M., 2008. Death after PEG: results of the National Confidential Enquiry into Patient Outcome and Death. *Gastrointestinal Endoscopy*, 68, pp. 223–7.

Légaré, F., Stacey, D., Gagnon, S., Dunn, S., Pluye, P., Kryworuchko, J. *et al.*, 2011. Validating a conceptual model for an inter-professional approach to shared decision making: a mixed methods study. *Journal of Evaluation in Clinical Practice*, 17, pp. 554–64.

Mackay, L., Morgan, A. and Bernstein, B., 2013. Factors affecting oral feeding with severe traumatic brain injury. *Journal of Head Trauma Rehabilitation*, 14, pp. 435–7.

Mitchell, S., Teno, J., Kiely, D., Shaffer, M., Jones, R., Prigerson, H. *et al.*, 2009. The clinical course of advanced dementia. *New England Journal of Medicine*, 361, pp. 1529–38.

NCCAC: National Collaborating Centre for Acute Care, 2006. *Nutrition support in adults: oral nutrition support, enteral tube feeding and parenteral nutrition: methods, evidence, guidance. Guidelines 32*. London: National Collaborating Centre for Acute Care.

RCP: Royal College of Physicians, 2010. *Oral feeding difficulties and dilemmas. A guide to practical care, particularly towards the end of life*. London: Royal College of Physicians.

Salzman, L., 2010. Rethinking guardianship (again) substituted decision-making as a violation for the integrations mandate of title II of the Americans with Disabilities Act. *University of Colorado Law Review*, 81, pp. 157–245.

Sessums, L., Zembrzuska, H. and Jackson, J., 2011. Does this patient have medical decision-making capacity? *JAMA*, 306, pp. 420–7.

Singer, P., Berger, M., Den-Berghe, G., Biolo, G., Calder, P., Forbes, A. *et al.*, 2009. ESPEN guidelines on parenteral nutrition: intensive care. *Clinical Nutrition*, 28, pp. 387–400.

UN: United Nations Convention on the Rights of Persons with Disabilities, 2006. *Final report of the Ad Hoc Committee on a Comprehensive and Integral International Convention on the Protection and Promotion of the Rights and Dignity of Persons with Disabilities*. Available through: <www.un.org/esa/socdev/enable/rights/ahcfinal repe.htm> [accessed 11 September 2015].

Weinberger, H., Cohen, J., Tadmor, B. and Singer, P., 2015. Towards a framework for untangling complexity: the interprofessional decision-making model for the complex patient. *Journal of the Association for Information Science and Technology*, 66, pp. 392–407.

WMA: World Medical Association Declaration of Helsinki, 1964. *Ethical principles for medical research involving human subjects*. Available through: <www.wma.net/ en/30publications/10policies/b3/> [accessed 11 September 2015].

10 Attitudinal, motivational and behavioural correlates of ethical leadership in healthcare teams

Martina Šendula-Pavelić, Zoran Sušanj and Ana Jakopec

Introduction

Competitive demands and the constant pressure for rapid technological, economic and organisational change and improvement have a profound impact on different company environments (Patzer and Voegtlin, 2012). Managing organisational change while maximising quality and economic profit without neglecting ethical principles, moral imperatives and professional standards set new demands on leaders' roles and responsibilities in all organisational settings, especially in healthcare institutions (Council of Europe, 1998).

The formation of professional identity, a complex process of integration of personal values and morals with professional standards, can only be achieved through interaction with other professionals. This interprofessional collaboration involves open communication about the professional roles and diverse experiences, as well as the consideration and exchange of different perspectives. Thinking and acting interprofessionally ultimately facilitates self-understanding as an essential part of professional identity, while improving healthcare outcomes. Contemporary changes in perspectives and approaches to healthcare and complex interprofessional work environment require empowered specialists who notice, raise and communicate ethical concerns in order to solve complex medical and ethical issues.

This leads to a renewed interest in research on ethical behaviour in healthcare settings and, especially, to the investigation of potential benefits of effective ethical leadership.

Ethical leadership is defined and measured differently, depending on the aspects of leadership the researchers consider to be crucial. Brown, Treviño and Harrison (2005) argue that ethical leaders are role models, and their integrity, honesty and fair treatment of employees encourage ethical behaviour within the organisation. They define ethical leadership as 'demonstration of normatively appropriate conduct through personal actions and interpersonal relations, and the promotion of such conduct among followers of two-way communication, reinforcement, and decision-making' (Brown *et al.*, 2005, p. 120). Mayer *et al.* (2009b) pointed out that leaders are vital for cultivating the ethical behaviour of their subordinates. In creating a fair environment, ethical executives encourage the ethical and prosocial behaviour of employees. Thus, research on ethical leadership investigates not only the perception of leaders' traits (for example, honesty), values (for example, altruism), and motivation (for example, power inhibition), but also leaders' behaviours (for example, fair and principled decision–making, intentional communication of ethical values and ethical guidance for their followers). Therefore, Yukl *et al.* (2011) point out four issues that appear most relevant to ethical leadership. These primarily include honesty and integrity, or consistency of actions with espoused values. In addition, behaviour intended to communicate or enforce ethical standards, fairness in decisions and the distribution of rewards (no favouritism or use of rewards to motivate improper behaviour), and behaviour that shows kindness, compassion and concern for the needs and feelings of others (rather than attempts to manipulate, abuse and exploit others for personal gain) are included. Thus, ethical leadership is not only about traits such as integrity and honesty, but also about efforts to make subordinates accountable for behaving ethically. Gini (1998) also describes ethical leaders as those who use their social power in their decisions, their own actions and their influence on others in such a way that they act in the best interests of followers and do not enact harm upon them by respecting the rights of all parties. Ethical leadership is, therefore, a means to sustain order and encourage the ethical conduct of followers.

In identifying antecedents of ethical leadership, researchers confirm important personality traits (Walumbwa and Schaubroeck, 2009; Kalshoven, Den Hartog and DeHoogh, 2011; Hoffman *et al.*, 2012) and virtues (Riggio *et al.*, 2010) of a leader behind the motivation for behaving ethically. Furthermore, a leader's moral identity (Mayer *et al.*, 2012), level of cognitive moral development (Schminke, Ambrose and Neubaum, 2005; McCauley *et al.*, 2006; Jordan *et al.*, 2013), ethical awareness (Resick *et al.*, 2006) and ethical role models that leaders had for learning ethical behaviour (Brown and Treviño, 2014) proved to be important predictors of ethical leadership.

Some researchers were interested in the process of developing and maintaining the ethical behaviour of leaders. These studies focus on the processes of (de)activation of moral self-regulatory mechanisms, variables that can explain what motivates managers and their followers to behave (un)ethically, the process of moral decision–making and the spillover effect in the workplace (Tenbrunsel and Smith-Crowe, 2008; Sharif and Scandura, 2014; Kluver, Frazier and Haidt, 2014).

The research identified various positive effects of ethical leadership. Employees who perceive their supervisor as ethical have more favourable job attitudes, such as job satisfaction (Piccolo *et al.*, 2010; Tanner *et al.*, 2010), commitment (Strobel, Tumasjan and Welpe, 2010), identification with the organisation (Walumbwa *et al.*, 2011) and trust (Van den Akker *et al.*, 2009). Ethical leadership is positively related to organisational citizenship behaviour (Mayer *et al.*, 2009b; Philipp and Lopez, 2013; Pitzer-Brandon, 2013), it reduces conflicts (Mayer *et al.*, 2012) and has a positive impact on the well-being of employees (Kalshoven and Boon, 2012). Ethical leaders support the climate in which employees feel free to report problems, and the ethical climate, in return, mediates the relationship between ethical leadership and employee misconduct, as well as some contextual and cultural factors that can strengthen the relationship between anticipated consequences of engaging in ethical leadership (Mayer, Kuenzi and Greenbaum, 2010; Vianello, Galliani and Haidt, 2010). Perhaps most importantly, employees' perceptions of ethical leadership predict their willingness to exert extra effort on the job and to report problems to management (Brown and Treviño, 2006).

Obviously, the outcomes of ethical leadership are beneficial for both organisation and employees. Most of the studies examined the individual outcomes of ethical leadership perceived, while they neglected outcomes that related to the employee perception of team functioning. Furthermore, to the best of our knowledge, the outcomes of ethical leadership have not been sufficiently investigated in healthcare organisations. Therefore, the primary objective of this study was to examine the relationship between healthcare team members' perception of the ethical leadership of their supervisors in relation to team members' attitudes and behaviours: work engagement, psychological empowerment, organisational citizenship behaviours, trust, perceived group effectiveness and cohesion in work teams, as a determinant of the relevant organisational outcomes in healthcare institutions.

Method

Participants

This research was conducted on a convenience sample of 169 members in non-managerial positions of 50 healthcare teams from 15 Croatian healthcare institutions (mainly hospitals and health centres). These were mostly inter-disciplinary teams consisting of both physicians and nurses. A clear hierarchical relationship was taken into account while choosing the sample: the team members were responsible to their immediate supervisor, and they had no formal authority over each other. Team members were interdependent while performing their tasks and shared a common (group) goal. Additionally, they had minimum team tenure of one-year duration. The gender composition of the sample was 72 per cent female and 57 per cent of team members were under 40 years old. Most of the team members (62 per cent) had more than six years of work experience. Additionally, more than half of the team members (52 per cent) had team tenure longer than six years. Moreover, 56 per cent of team members were academically educated.

Instruments and procedure

This research was conducted in the team members' institutions. Participation in the study was confidential and voluntary. Team members completed a questionnaire, which took them approximately 25 minutes. This unique questionnaire consisted of multiple scales, including the following:

- The Ethical Leadership Questionnaire (adapted from Yukl *et al.*, 2011) contains 15 items and captured team members' assessment of their leaders' ethical behaviour (example item: 'Our superior communicates clear ethical standards for members').
- The Organisational Citizenship Behaviour Scale (adapted from Lee and Allen, 2002) consists of three subscales (eight items each) measuring the organisational citizenship behaviour of team members toward organisation (example item: 'The members of my team defend the organisation when other employees criticise it'), supervisor (example item: 'The members of my team help the supervisor in performing duties') and peers (example item: 'The members of my team help each other in performing their duties').
- The Team Empowerment Questionnaire (adapted from Kirkman *et al.*, 2004), as a set of cognitions shaped by work environment, consists of 12 items and measures the potency, meaningfulness, autonomy and impact of team members (example item: 'My team feels that its tasks are worthwhile').
- The Team Work Engagement Questionnaire (adapted from Torrente *et al.*, 2012a) consists of nine items and measures a team's vigour, dedication and absorption (example item: 'My team is proud of the work that we do').
- The Organisational Trust Inventory (adapted from Nyhan and Marlowe, 1997) includes eight items measuring the team members' trust in leadership (example item: 'My team members believe that our supervisor is technically competent at the critical elements of the job') and four items measuring the team members' trust in organisation (example item: 'My team members believe that the organisation will treat us fairly').
- The Perceived Group Performance Questionnaire (adapted from Jung and Sosik, 2002) consists of five items measuring a work group's perceived effectiveness (example item: 'My group is effective in meeting task requirements').
- The Cohesion in Work Teams Questionnaire (adapted from Carless and De Paola, 2000) consists of ten items and measured the team members' task cohesion, social cohesion and individual attraction to the group (example item: 'Our team would like to spend time together outside of work hours').

All the items were presented in a Likert type of format with a scale ranging from 1 = strongly disagree to 5 = completely agree. A composite score was defined as a mean value of all item estimations for each scale.

Results

Results of the correlational analysis are presented in Table 10.1.

Table 10.1 Descriptive statistics and correlations of all variables measured

	N	M	SD	1	2	3	4	5	6	7	8	9	10
1. EL	150	3.87	.73	.91	.53	.58	.43	.58	.50	.84	.58	.43	.42
2. OCBO	161	3.99	.65		.83	.55	.64	.66	.62	.43	.73	.45	.50
3. OCBS	166	3.70	.64			.72	.53	.52	.47	.48	.51	.31	.35
4. OCBP	158	4.01	.55				.73	.66	.61	.46	.71	.55	.37
5. PE	161	3.97	.44					.68	.68	.54	.64	.70	.36
6. WE	162	3.84	.63						.79	.43	.62	.54	.52
7. TL	163	4.00	.74							.88	.52	.35	.28
8. TO	165	3.88	.75								.68	.48	.35
9. PGP	166	4.28	.57									.77	.38
10. GC	160	3.45	.64										.69

Note: All correlations are statistically significant ($p < .001$). Cronbach alpha coefficients are presented on the diagonal. EL = Ethical Leadership; OCBO = Organisational Citizenship Behaviour toward Organisation; OCBS = Organisational Citizenship Behaviour toward Supervisor; OCBP = Organisational Citizenship Behaviour toward Peers; PE = Psychological Empowerment; WE = Work Engagement; TL = Trust in Leadership; TO = Trust in Organisation; PGP = Perceived Group Performance; GC = Group Cohesiveness.

Ethical leadership is positively correlated with all the team members' desirable attitudinal, motivational and behavioural outcomes. Specifically, team members who consider their leader as ethical exhibit higher levels of organisational citizenship behaviours, especially toward their supervisor, as well as toward organisation and peers. More precisely, they (1) help their peers and supervisor when absent and in situations where they have work- or non-work-related problems; (2) assist others with their duties; (3) share personal property with both their supervisor and peers; (4) show concern and courtesy toward their peers and supervisor, even under the most trying (business or personal) situations; and (5) adjust their work schedule to the other employees' requests for time off. At the same time, for instance, they try to keep up with developments in the organisation, express loyalty to the organisation, demonstrate concern about the organisation's image and show pride when representing their organisation. These team members are also empowered and engaged in their work. In other words, they believe that they can be effective in performing their duties, their tasks are important and valuable, they experience substantial freedom, independence and discretion in their work, and they produce significant and important work for the organisation. Additionally, they have high levels of energy, persistence, resilience and the willingness to invest effort in performing their duties, they feel enthusiastic and proud about their job and feel happily immersed in their work. In addition, team members that perceive their leader as ethical tend to have higher levels of trust in leadership and the organisation. Moreover, these team members perceive their team as efficient and cohesive.

Discussion

This chapter attempts to contribute to the understanding of the role of ethical leadership in healthcare institutions and healthcare teams. We found that members of healthcare teams perceive ethical leadership and that the latter had moderate to strong positive correlations with the attitudes, motivation and behaviour of their team.

As expected, the perception of the supervisors' ethical leadership is most correlated with trust in leadership and the organisation. The main objective of a leader's behaviour and effective leadership is to influence the activities and behaviour of their employees in achieving organisational goals. If the supervisor is seen to be ethical, then his actions have credibility and organisational goals can be realised. Trust relationships in the workplace affect intrinsic motivation for providing effective healthcare (Gilson, Palmer and Schneider, 2005). The higher levels of trust in healthcare settings are related to lower surveillance and a better quality of health services. Based on the systematic review of articles reporting research findings on workplace trust relationships and motivation of healthcare workers, Okello and Gilson (2015) found that workplace relationships that are supportive and respectful have a positive influence on healthcare workers' performance, quality of healthcare service and intention to stay in the organisation.

Team members who consider their leader to be ethical also indicate higher levels of organisational citizenship behaviours, especially toward their supervisor, as well as toward their organisation and co-workers. Organisational citizenship behaviour is not imposed by the work role, but is behaviour 'behind the role' and a matter of the personal choice of the individual and their emotional connection with the organisation. Those behaviours are associated with a number of important outcomes for both the team and the organisation. These outcomes include measures of profitability, performance, service quality and customer satisfaction. The employee motivated intrinsically will behave responsibly toward the organisation. Affective loyalty to the supervisor, which is perceived as ethical, can strengthen the intrinsically driven prosocial motivation of employees and encourage greater investment of effort and perseverance at work (Grant, 2008). Studies confirmed the importance of how employees perceive their leader's behaviour and whether the leader 'walks the talk' and communicates ethical values and responsibilities. If the values of altruism, compassion, honesty and fairness are not recognised in a leader's behaviour, then it may contribute to higher levels of employee deviance. Furthermore, inconsistency of behaviour concerning the values that the supervisor stands for can be perceived as supervisor hypocrisy (Treviño, Hartman and Brown, 2000; Simons, 2002; Mayer *et al.*, 2009a). This explains the importance of assessing the ethics of a supervisor's behaviour and the influence they can have on the quality of healthcare (Bedi, Alpaslan and Green, 2015).

Ethical leadership is positively related to the team empowerment perceived. Empowered teams have a collective belief that they can be effective, their tasks are important to the organisation, their job is valuable and worthwhile, and they have freedom, independence and discretion in their work (Kirkman *et al.*, 2004). In the context of healthcare services, only empowered healthcare teams can make timely and prompt decisions that can sometimes save lives. This can result in improved healthcare outcomes for individuals and communities by delivering high-quality healthcare service and minimising risks and harm to patients.

Perceived ethical leadership is positively correlated with the work engagement of the team. Teamwork engagement, characterised by a high level of energy, dedication and absorption of the team members in doing their job (Torrente *et al.*, 2012a), ensures appropriate, expedient and effective interprofessional healthcare service. Teamwork engagement contributes positively to the experience of self-efficacy, the positive emotional state of the team and the success of the working team in general (Salanova *et al.*, 2003; Bakker, van Emmerik and Euwema, 2006; Torrente *et al.*, 2012b). The organisational benefits of effective teamwork in healthcare settings are usually described as reduced hospitalisation time and costs, fewer unanticipated admissions, better patient accessibility and improved coordination of care. Team-level benefits include efficient utilisation of services, enhanced communication and maximal diversity of professional expertise. Engaged team members report enhanced job satisfaction, greater role clarity and enhanced well-being (Mickan, 2005). Finally, patients of engaged healthcare teams report enhanced satisfaction, awareness of treatment and improved health outcomes.

The experiences of the cohesiveness of healthcare practitioners within teams are important. Team spirit that is generated by working together over time, meaning perceived team efficacy, cohesion, shared enjoyment and pride in their achievements, has direct consequences on patient care. Cohesive teams are effective teams. Employees build up a sense of commitment, trust and mutual respect through participation in team tasks, a team spirit that is reinforced with ethical leadership (Mickan and Rodger, 2005). Ethical leadership helps create and strengthen the climate of trust and cohesion in healthcare teams. Ethical leaders support the climate in which employees feel free to report problems and this is a predictor of group-level helping behaviour in the organisation (Cruess, Cruess and Steinert, 2008; Kalshoven and Boon, 2012). Developing climates that encourage ethical behaviour is important, especially in healthcare settings, because it is positively related to all relevant organisational outcomes that have direct consequences for the provision of medical care.

There are some study limitations that should be addressed. First, the cross-sectional design of this study does not allow one to infer causality. Furthermore, the measures that we applied to a smaller number of the healthcare teams are not context-specific. It would be worthwhile adapting them in further research so that they measure, for example, concrete behaviours that outline team-specific performance relevant for hospital settings. In addition, further research should include some other variables associated with social and physical distance that we did not consider. It would also be worthwhile to include the supervisors' perceived ethical behaviour, as well as to detect possible discrepancies between the supervisors' self-assessment of their ethical behaviour and the same behaviour perceived by their subordinates.

Conclusion

The way in which followers perceive ethical leadership has direct consequences on their work performance (Greenbaum, Mawritz and Piccolo, 2015). Only effective interprofessional teamwork can address the complex medical needs of the patients and enhance the quality of patient care (Borrill *et al.* 2000). The American Board of Internal Medicine (ABIM, 1995) and the Association of American Medical Colleges listed nine behaviours necessary for physicians to exhibit in order to meet their obligations to patients, communities and their profession. Being a professional and behaving like one is about delivering services to an appropriately high standard, with the knowledge and skills learnt, to deliver care with morality and integrity. The identification of teams with a lower level of desired work and organisational attitudes, motivation and behaviours, and engaging the teams in activities designed to raise the level may bring about better patient care. It, therefore, seems worthwhile to engage in raising the awareness of the consequences of ethical leadership in healthcare settings. This can be achieved primarily by conducting training programmes to empower the healthcare managers with ethical leadership, as well as through other human resource development activities that promote ethical competence in interprofessional collaborative healthcare teams.

Healthcare professionalism is a complex multidimensional concept described in terms of integrity, respect, compassion, altruism, accountability, excellence, duty, service, honour and respect for others. Practising medicine demands a strong commitment to professional excellence that incorporates ethics (Huddle, 2005; Birden *et al.*, 2013). Healthcare institutions should strive to ensure ethical leadership and an ethical climate by educating and training their supervisors, and by recruitment and professional selection of healthcare workers for supervisory positions. As Brown and Treviño (2006) recommended, healthcare institutions can use four approaches to attract and then encourage, support and further develop ethical leadership: selection, role modelling, training, and organisational culture and socialisation. Our results show that healthcare teams need ethical leaders. All healthcare workers at all organisational levels regularly face difficult choices and challenges where their integrity and ethics are tested. Enhancing ethical behaviour within healthcare institutions and emphasising the intrinsically rewarding aspects of the work rooted in the definition of a medical professional is required. This is especially relevant in the contemporary demanding climate and circumstances of discontent of both healthcare workers and patients with the growing social problems, inability to articulate a claim by profession, insufficient funding, and so on. Unless leaders model and guide employees' behaviours and promote ethics within a professional organisation's agenda and, further, through the entire healthcare system, the employees will not internalise the meaning of the code of ethics and the ethical delivery of healthcare services will be questioned (Ogunfowora, 2014).

In conclusion, continued development of sensibility for ethical leadership within healthcare institutions is needed. Stronger involvement of interprofessional collaboration within hospital settings (Martina *et al.*, 2010; WHO, 2010) will bring significant improvement in outcomes following interventions based on interprofessional collaboration. There is a growing demand for research to find predictors of effective healthcare teams and for applied research to guide leadership practice. Psychology research, counselling and professional expertise can contribute to the clarification of the ethical responsibility of the leadership of healthcare institutions and improve the ethical competence of healthcare personnel, developing bioethical sensibility. Bioethics calls for the interdisciplinary approach and ethical methodologies. Strong ethical healthcare professionals, teams and organisations as a whole can be guaranteed only by recognising the need for ethical leadership, training and cultivating leadership expertise as a significant part of professional competence.

References

ABIM: American Board of Internal Medicine Committee on Evaluation of Clinical Competence, 1995. *Project professionalism*. Philadelphia, PA: American Board of Internal Medicine.

Bakker, A.B., van Emmerik, H. and Euwema, M.C., 2006. Crossover of burnout and engagement in work teams. *Work and Occupations*, 33, pp. 464–89.

Bedi, A., Alpaslan, C.M. and Green, S., 2015. A meta-analytic review of ethical leadership outcomes and moderators. *Journal of Business Ethics*, pp. 1–20. Available through: <www.academia.edu/12098293/A_Meta-analytic_Review_of_Ethical_Leadership_Outcomes_and_Moderators> [accessed 12 September 2015].

Birden, H., Glass, N., Wilson, I., Harrison, M., Usherwood, T. and Nass, D., 2013. Defining professionalism in medical education: a Best Evidence Medical Education (BEME) systematic review. *Medical Teacher*, 35, pp. 1252–66.

Borrill, C., West, M., Shapiro, D. and Rees, A., 2000. Team working and effectiveness in health care. *British Journal of Healthcare Management*, 6, pp. 364–71.

Brown, M.E. and Treviño, L.K., 2006. Ethical leadership: a review and future directions. *Leadership Quarterly*, 17, pp. 595–616.

Brown, M.E. and Treviño, L.K., 2014. Do role models matter? An investigation of role modelling as an antecedent of perceived ethical leadership. *Journal of Business Ethics*, 122, pp. 587–98.

Brown, M.E., Treviño, L.K. and Harrison, D.A., 2005. Ethical leadership: a social learning perspective for construct development and testing. *Organisational Behaviour and Human Decision Processes*, 97, pp. 117–34.

Carless, S.A. and De Paola, C., 2000. The measurement of cohesion in work teams. *Small Group Research*, 31, pp. 107–18.

Council of Europe, 1998. *The development and implementation of quality improvement systems (QIS) in health care – Recommendation No. R (97) 17 and explanatory memorandum.* Strasbourg: Council of Europe.

Cruess, S.R., Cruess, R.L. and Steinert, Y., 2008. Role modelling – making the most of a powerful teaching strategy. *British Medical Journal*, 336, pp. 718–21.

Gilson, L., Palmer, N. and Schneider, H., 2005. Trust and health worker performance: exploring a conceptual framework using South African evidence. *Social Science and Medicine*, 61, pp. 1418–29.

Gini, A., 1998. Moral leadership and business ethics. In: J.B. Ciulla ed., *Ethics, the heart of leadership*. Westport, CT: Quorum Books, pp. 27–45.

Grant, A.M., 2008. Does intrinsic motivation fuel the prosocial fire? Motivational synergy in predicting persistence, performance, and productivity. *Journal of Applied Psychology*, 93, p. 48.

Greenbaum, R.L., Mawritz, M.B. and Piccolo, R.F., 2015. When leaders fail to 'walk the talk': supervisor undermining and perceptions of leader hypocrisy. *Journal of Management*, 41, pp. 929–56.

Hoffman, B.J., Strang, S., Kuhnert, K., Campbell, K., Kennedy, K. and Lopilato, A., 2012. Leader narcissism and ethical context: effects on ethical leadership and leader effectiveness. *Journal of Leadership and Organisational Studies*, 20, pp. 25–37.

Huddle, T.S., 2005. Viewpoint: teaching professionalism: is medical morality a competency? *Academic Medicine*, 80, pp. 885–91.

Jordan, J., Brown, M.E., Treviño, L.K. and Finkelstein, S., 2013. Someone to look up to: executive–follower ethical reasoning and perceptions of ethical leadership. *Journal of Management*, 39, pp. 660–83.

Jung, D. and Sosik, J.J., 2002. Transformational leadership in work groups. The role of empowerment, cohesiveness, and collective-efficacy on perceived group performance. *Small Group Research*, 33, pp. 313–36.

Kalshoven, K. and Boon, C.T., 2012. Ethical leadership, employee well-being and helping: the moderating role of human resource management. *Journal of Personnel Psychology*, 11, pp. 60–68.

Kalshoven, K., Den Hartog, D. and De Hoogh, A., 2011. Ethical leader behavior and big five factors of personality. *Journal of Business Ethics*, 100, pp. 349–66.

Kirkman, B.L., Rosem, B., Tesluk, P.E. and Gibson, C.B., 2004. The impact of team empowerment on virtual team performance: the moderating role of face-to-face interaction. *Academy of Management Journal*, 47, pp. 175–92.

Kluver, J., Frazier, R. and Haidt, J., 2014. Behavioral ethics for Homo economicus, Homo heuristicus, and Homo duplex. *Organisational Behavior and Human Decision Processes*, 123, pp. 150–8.

Lee, K. and Allen, N.J., 2002. Organisational citizenship behavior and workplace deviance: the role of affect and cognitions. *Journal of Applied Psychology*, 87, p. 131.

Martina, J.S., Ummenhoferb, W., Manserc, T. and Spiriga, R., 2010. Inter-professional collaboration among nurses and physicians: making a difference in patient outcome. *Swiss Medical Weekly*, 140, pp. w13062.

Mayer, D.M., Aquino, K., Greenbaum, R.L. and Kuenzi, M., 2012. Who displays ethical leadership and why does it matter? An examination of antecedents and consequences of ethical leadership. *Academy of Management Journal*, 55, pp. 151–71.

Mayer, D.M., Kuenzi, M. and Greenbaum, R.L., 2010. Examining the link between ethical leadership and employee misconduct: the mediating role of ethical climate. *Journal of Business Ethics*, 95, pp. 7–16.

Mayer, D.M., Brown, M., Priesemuth, M. and Kuenzi, M., 2009a. Antecedents and consequences of employee-supervisor agreement on ethical leadership. *Proceedings of the annual meeting of the Academy of Management*, Chicago.

Mayer, D.M., Kuenzi, M., Greenbaum, R.L., Bardes, M. and Salvador, R., 2009b. How does ethical leadership flow? Test of a trickle-down model. *Organisational Behavior and Human Decision Processes*, 108, pp. 1–13.

McCauley, C.D., Drath, W.H., Palus, C.J., O'Connor, P.M.G. and Baker, B., 2006. The use of constructive-developmental theory to advance the understanding of leadership. *Leadership Quarterly*, 17, pp. 634–53.

Mickan, S.M., 2005. Evaluating the effectiveness of health care teams. *Australian Health Review*, 29, pp. 211–17.

Mickan, S.M. and Rodger, S.A., 2005. Effective health care teams: a model of six characteristics developed from shared perceptions. *Journal of Inter-professional Care*, 19, pp. 358–70.

Nyhan, R.C. and Marlowe, H.A., 1997. Development and psychometric properties of the organisational trust inventory. *Evaluation Review*, 21, pp. 614–35.

Ogunfowora, B., 2014. It's all a matter of consensus: leader role modelling strength as a moderator of the links between ethical leadership and employee outcomes. *Human Relations*, pp. 1–24.

Okello, D.R.O. and Gilson, L., 2015. Exploring the influence of trust relationships on motivation in the health sector: a systematic review. *Human Resources for Health*, 13, pp. 1–18.

Patzer, M. and Voegtlin, C., 2012. Leadership ethics and organisational change: sketching the field. University of Zurich, Institute of Organisation and Administrative Science (IOU), *IOU Working Paper Series No. 113*. Available through SSRN: <http://ssrn.com/abstract=1701002> [accessed 13 September 2015].

Philipp, B.L.U. and Lopez, P.D.J., 2013. The moderating role of ethical leadership: investigating relationships among employee psychological contracts, commit-ment, and citizenship behavior. *Journal of Leadership & Organizational Studies*, 20, pp. 304–15.

Piccolo, R.F., Greenbaum, R., Den Hartog, D.N. and Folger, R., 2010. The relationship between ethical leadership and core job characteristics. *Journal of Organisational Behavior*, 31, pp. 259–78.

Pitzer-Brandon, D.M., 2013. *The impact of ethical leadership on employee organisational citizenship behaviors*. Ph.D. Capella University. Available through: <http://gradworks.umi.com/3603790.pdf> [accessed 13 September 2015].

Resick, C.J., Hanges, P.J., Dickson, M.W. and Mitchelson, J.K., 2006. A cross-cultural examination of the endorsement of ethical leadership. *Journal of Business Ethics*, 63, pp. 345–59.

Riggio, R.E., Zhu, W., Reina, C. and Maroosis, J.A., 2010. Virtue-based measurement of ethical leadership: The Leadership Virtues Questionnaire. *Consulting Psychology Journal: Practice and Research*, 62, pp. 235–50.

Salanova, M., Llorens, S., Cifre, E., Martínez, I.M. and Schaufeli, W.B., 2003. Perceived collective efficacy, subjective well-being and task performance among electronic work groups: an experimental study. *Small Group Research*, 34, pp. 43–73.

Schminke, M., Ambrose, M. and Neubaum, D., 2005. The effect of leader moral development on ethical climate and employee attitudes. *Organisational Behaviour and Human Decisions Processes*, 97, pp. 135–51.

Sharif, M.M. and Scandura, T.A., 2014. Moral identity: linking ethical leadership to follower decision making. In: L. Neider and C. Schriesheim eds., *Advances in authentic and ethical leadership*. Research in Management, Volume 10. Charlotte, NC: Information Age Publishing.

Simons,T., 2002. Behavioral integrity: the perceived alignment between managers' words and deeds as a research focus. *Organisation Science*, 13, pp. 18–35.

Strobel, M., Tumasjan, A. and Welpe, I., 2010. Do business ethics pay off? The influence of ethical leadership on organisational attractiveness. *Journal of Psychology*, 218, pp. 213–24.

Tanner, C., Brugger, A., van Schie, S. and Lebherz, C. (2010). Actions speak louder than words: the benefits of ethical behaviors of leaders. *Journal of Psychology*, 218, pp. 225–33.

Tenbrunsel, A.E. and Smith-Crowe, K., 2008. Ethical decision making: where we've been and where we're going. *The Academy of Management Annals*, 2, pp. 545–607.

Torrente, P., Salanova, M., Llorens, S. and Schaufeli, W.B., 2012a. From I to we: the factorial validity of a team work engagement scale. In: S.P. Gonçalves and J.G. Neves eds., *Occupational health psychology: from burnout to well-being*. Lisbon, Portugal: Edições Sílabo.

Torrente, P., Salanova, M., Llorens, S. and Schaufeli, W.B., 2012b. Teams make it work: how team work engagement mediates between social resources and performance in teams. *Psicothema*, 24, pp. 106–12.

Treviño, L.K., Hartman, L.P. and Brown, M.E., 2000. Moral person and moral manager: how executives develop a reputation for ethical leadership. *California Management Review*, 42, pp. 128–42.

Van den Akker, L., Heres, L., Lausthuizen, K. and Six, F., 2009. Ethical leadership and trust: it's all about meeting expectations. *International Journal of Leadership Studies*, 5, pp. 102–22.

Vianello, M., Galliani, E.M. and Haidt, J., 2010. Elevation at work: the organisational effects of leaders' moral excellence. *Journal of Positive Psychology*, 5, pp. 390–411.

Walumbwa, F.O. and Schaubroeck, J., 2009. Leader personality traits and employee voice behavior: mediating roles of ethical leadership and work group psychological safety. *Journal of Applied Psychology*, 94, pp. 1275–86.

Walumbwa, F.O., Mayer, D.M., Wang, P., Wang, H., Workman, K. and Christensen, A.L., 2011. Linking ethical leadership to employee performance: the roles of leader-member exchange, self-efficacy, and organisational identification. *Organisational Behavior and Human Decision Processes*, 115, pp. 204–13.

WHO: World Health Organization (2010). *Framework for action on inter-professional education and collaborative practice*. Geneva, WHO, 2010. Available through: <www.who.int/hrh/resources/framework_action/en/> [accessed 13 September 2015].

Yukl, G., Mahsud, R., Hassan, S. and Prussia, G.E., 2011. An improved measure of ethical leadership. *Journal of Leadership & Organizational Studies*, 20, pp. 1–11.

11 Cooperation between managers and the medical profession in the context of strategic decision-making in non-profit hospitals

A manageable challenge?

Stephanie Rüsch

Introduction

The healthcare system constitutes an essential part of both German society and its economy. Health expenditure in Germany amounted to more than 300 billion euros in 2013, accounting for approximately 11 per cent of the gross domestic profit (Federal Statistical Office, 2015a). Hospitals represent the major healthcare providers among the healthcare services. From the 300 billion euros expenditure on health, almost 80 billion euros were spent on the hospital market (Federal Statistical Office, 2015b). Due to this considerable amount of expenditure, the hospital market forms one of the main targets for cost-reducing measures induced by the government.

One of the distinctive features of the hospital market is its regulatory nature, meaning that the state influences the market considerably through laws and regulations. These regulations have undergone significant changes in the last decade which aim at increasing the efficiency of medical service providers. One major aspect in this context is the hospital funding system. The German hospital funding system allowed full compensation of treatment costs up to the 1990s. However, since the mandatory introduction of the diagnosis-related group system in 2004, hospitals' refunds are based on fixed amounts for specific medical diagnoses. Any costs that exceed this amount are not refunded by the system. The primary aim of this reform was to reduce overcapacity, increase economic efficiency and foster transparency. Another implication was the enhancement of competition between the hospitals (Schreyögg, Tiemann and Busse, 2006). As a result, numerous hospitals have been closed down and others have adopted competitive strategies in order to react to the changing conditions of the hospital market (Bazzoli, 2004). Hence, the adequate management of hospitals has become imperative to their survival in this dynamic environment.

In addition to these challenges induced by the external environment, hospitals struggle with tensions between internal actors at the organisational level.

This appears to be true not only for the interaction between medical and nursing staff, but also for the relationship between the medical profession and the hospital managers. From the perspective of organisational theory, the hospital represents an exceptional object of investigation due to its tripartite structure (management, medical and nursing staff) and resulting relationships between internal actors. A prominent approach to classify this particular organisational form has been put forward by Mintzberg (1980), who describes the hospital configuration as a 'professional bureaucracy'. Studies that investigate the relationships between internal actors in the hospital setting have found that physicians tend to react with resistance to managerial attempts to constrain and control their medical actions (e.g. Anderson and McDaniel, 2000). Remarkably, studies investigating the relationship between the medical profession and managers have so far focused mostly on the medical profession (e.g. Kuhlmann *et al.*, 2013), whereas literature on the interaction between medical staff and management from the managers' point of view is scarce.

Taking this research gap into account, this chapter investigates the potentially conflictual relationship between hospital managers and the medical profession from the managers' point of view on the basis of a field study in 13 German non-profit hospitals. More specifically, the purpose is to provide answers to the following research questions:

1   How do hospital managers perceive the role of the medical profession in the context of strategic decision-making?
2   How do hospital managers interact with the medical profession within the process of strategic planning, implementation and control?

Exploring this topic is of particular interest for the following reasons: first, as indicated above, the managerial point of view regarding their relationship to the medical profession has not yet been adequately addressed. However, insights into the managers' motives and perceptions related to this topic could increase mutual understanding to the advantage of cooperative work within the hospital. As studies have shown, cooperation between managers and physicians is crucial to the survival of the hospital organisation itself (Garelick, 2005).

Literature review and conceptual framework

One of the peculiarities distinguishing German hospitals from other organisations is its tripartite vertical authority hierarchy. Correspondingly, the board of managers involves the administrative director (who usually acts as the chief executive officer, CEO, at the same time), the medical director and the director of nursing (e.g. Rohde, 1962; Wilkesmann, 2009). Remarkably, the core processes within the hospital (medical treatment) require particular expert knowledge exclusively obtained by the medical profession. Resulting from this information asymmetry, neither the managers – including the CEO – nor the nursing staff are able to assess the quality and efficiency of the healthcare service. Mintzberg (1980) classifies this organisational configuration, in which the operative processes represent the essential part of the value creation processes, as professional bureaucracy (see Figure 11.1). The predominance of highly qualified staff who work in the core processes (*operating core*) and who possess considerable power due to a high degree of decentralisation are characteristic of this organisational type. The management, by contrast, forms the *strategic apex* of the organisation. Its primary task is to support the operating core by conducting negotiations with external parties and by ensuring the provision of the resources required to the professionals. The *support staff* is concerned with rather routine work in order to back up the professionals in the operating core. The *technostructure*, which sees to the formalisation and control of the organisational processes, remains minimal in this organisation type, since the output of the professionals cannot easily be standardised.

Studies investigating the reaction of the medical profession to the introduction of regulatory measures in the hospital setting underline the considerable conflict potential between the managerial and the medical concerns (e.g. Morgan and Ogbonna, 2008; Fiol, Pratt and O'Connor, 2009). In this context, the medical profession is characterised by their notable efforts to maintain autonomy, encouraged by the decentralised organisational structure inherent in a professional bureaucracy which transfers considerable power to the professionals working in the *operating core* of the organisation (Numerato, Salvatore and Fattore, 2012). According to the logic of the professional bureaucracy, managers are perceived rather as administrators responsible for support activities, such as allocating resources to the experts who use them to fulfil the major objective of the hospital: providing healthcare services. Even strategic initiatives, which traditionally belong to the area of authority of the management, can emanate from the medical profession rather than the managers themselves (Mintzberg, 2010). Thus, managerial attempts to regulate and control the medical actions in order to align them to strategic goals can provoke extensive resistance among the professionals who perceive such measures to be a threat to their professional identity (e.g. Walter and Lopez, 2008; Boonstra

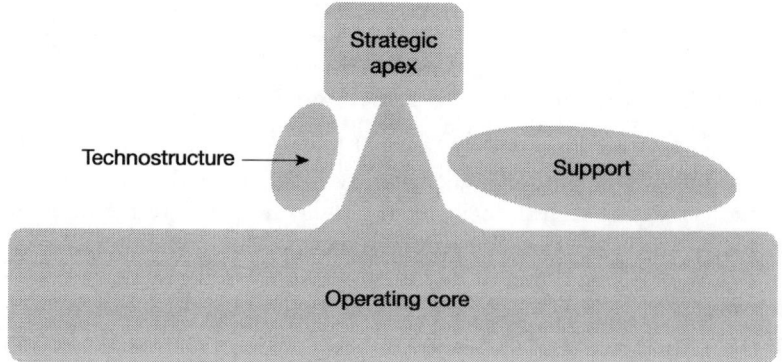

Figure 11.1 Professional bureaucracy according to Mintzberg (1980)

and Broekhuis, 2010; Numerato *et al.*, 2012). In light of the physicians' power within the hospital, such indications of resistance contribute to the notion of 'professional control' (Freidson, 2001) as a third logic next to the managerial and market controls. However, in the course of the increasing economisation of hospitals, it has been argued that a shift in power toward the management has occurred (e.g. Scott, 1993; Bär, 2011), since the physicians have become more dependent on managers who possess the knowledge to cope with the emerging economic requirements. Studies focusing on finding solutions to alleviate the conflicts between the professional and the managerial culture recommend the integration of these two worlds by reorganising hospital structures and fostering teamwork. This can be achieved through a compromise between bureaucratising professionals and professionalising managers (Lega and Pietro, 2005). In order to establish adequate structures for this purpose, insights into the relationship between physicians and managers are required.

Methodology

The data from this study was based on exploratory semi-structured expert interviews which were conducted within the frame of a dissertation project.[1] The sample consists of 13 managers of Christian non-profit hospitals in leading managerial positions (see Table 11.1). The size of the hospitals varies from small (fewer than 300 beds) to large (more than 600 beds). Furthermore, they differ in terms of location (urban and rural).

The interview guidelines were intentionally kept broad and open in order to match the exploratory nature of the methodology. Topics to be addressed

Table 11.1 Sample

Hospital no.	Hospital size	Location	Position of respondent	Duration of interview (minutes)
1	small	urban	adm. director	17
2	medium	urban	CEO	31
3	small	urban	adm. director	35
4	medium	urban	CEO	54
5	large	urban	CEO	28
6	medium	urban	CEO	61
7	medium	rural	adm. director	23
8	medium	urban	CEO	79
9	small	urban	CEO	77
10	medium	urban	CEO	57
11	large	urban	CEO	31
12	medium	rural	CEO	30
13	medium	rural	CEO	28

included the strategic direction of the hospital, determinants of the strategy and strategic planning, and implementation processes, by means of performance measurement and incentive systems. The interviews were digitally recorded and transcribed in compliance with the respondents' permission. Subsequently, the interview material was analysed by qualitative content analysis (Mayring, 2000) regarding the managers' perception of the medical profession and the interaction between managers and physicians within the scope of strategy-making.

Results

How hospital managers perceive the medical profession

According to the statements in the data, managers perceive the physicians as powerful actors within the organisation. This power apparently stems from various circumstances which will be explained in the following.

The primary source of the physicians' power seems to arise from their medical knowledge which constitutes an information advantage vis-à-vis the managers and, thus, contributes to their position as professional experts within the organisation. This corresponds to the power of the *operating core* in Mintzberg's (1980) professional bureaucracy. Accordingly, Expert (Exp.) 10 mentions that it would not be reasonable for him as a manager to set priorities when pondering potential directions to enhance their medical service offer. In fact, the chief physicians are closer to the medical developments in their specialist fields, so they are in charge of indicating promising opportunities (Exp. 12). Apart from their knowledge advantage, chief physicians are considered to be important 'marketing factors' (Exp. 9) with regard to attracting personnel and patients. Exp. 3, for instance, explains that recruitment depends to a great extent on the leadership skills of the chief physicians. Having a competent chief physician as a kind of 'flagship' (Exp. 7) constitutes a considerable advantage, particularly regarding the recruitment of specialists. Furthermore, Exp. 2 states that he publishes the benchmark results of the chief physicians in comparison to their counterparts from competing hospitals in order to demonstrate the quality of his hospital. Correspondingly, the overall reputation of the hospital benefits from the success of its chief physicians. Another source of power stems from the substantial shortage of doctors in Germany and, hence, the physicians' freedom in selecting the hospital in which they prefer to work. Hospitals, especially in rural areas, however, face difficulties with regard to attracting personnel (Exp. 10). Concerning personal attributes, chief physicians are considered to be 'highly autonomy-seeking' and rather 'self-confident' (Exp. 8) with respect to the manner in which they lead their departments.

From the managers' point of view, certain conflicts can arise within their relationship to the medical profession. First, the conflicting interests between economics, on the one hand, and the quality of medical care, on the other hand, still constitute a major topic of discussion. Exp. 4, for example, states that the chief physicians argue that the optimal quality of care should have the highest priority, whereas he reasons that the economic survival of the hospital should be the primary objective:

> The chief physicians always talk about optimal patient care, but I said this is not true. (. . .) Maintaining the system. That is my primary objective. Optimal patient care and the maintenance of the system can work against one another. I can rapidly go bankrupt with optimal patient care.
>
> (Exp. 4)

In this context, Exp. 8 argues that there is not necessarily any ethical conflict between medical and economic objectives, because both concepts oppose the waste of resources.

However, this sort of conflict appears to be alleviated under certain circumstances. From the managers' point of view, the 'economic understanding' (Exp. 3) of chief physicians contributes to reducing conflicts. Physicians, for instance, who have studied economic subjects in the course of their academic career seem to have less difficulty relating to economic reasoning. Accordingly, hospital managers with a dual educational background (e.g. business studies as a second degree in addition to medical study) help to build a bridge between the managerial and professional worlds (Exp. 3).

How hospital managers interact with the medical profession

As indicated above, managers depend on the physicians' expert knowledge in order to lead the hospital in an adequate way. Hence, in spite of the centralised hierarchical organisation structure, which is inherent in the hospital setting, there is a strong need for the managers to ensure the physicians' commitment. Managing an organisation requires the use of several instruments with regard to aligning the members of the organisation toward a common strategy. Among these are incentive systems which aim at encouraging desirable actions, but also restricting instruments geared toward the avoidance of undesirable actions. In this respect, the interaction between the managers and the medical profession will be illuminated from the managerial point of view in the following.

One of the managers' major concerns appears to be the involvement of the physicians in the strategy–making process. Accordingly, the managers expect the chief physicians to contribute to the strategic planning by searching for potential opportunities regarding the development of their departments, making suggestions for new specialised interdisciplinary departments and coming up with ideas regarding changes in the organisational structure or pro-cesses. Exp. 12, for instance, states that his chief physicians are encouraged to monitor market trends and show potentials for the development of their medical department: 'This is something we expect from our chief physicians (. . .). That they observe the development of medical services outside of our hospital and signal where the gaps are in our services, and should we implement interdisciplinary cooperation or centre?'

Furthermore, the physicians are involved in investment decisions regarding new medical equipment or facilities (Exp. 2). Apparently, the managers depend on the medical know-how of the medical profession in order to conduct well-founded strategic planning and consider potential for innovations. In this regard, all respondent managers mentioned that there should be a balance between bottom-up and top-down decision-making: on the one hand, the chief physicians contribute their ideas and give recommendations based on their professional know-how; on the other hand, managers need to assess the feasibility of these suggestions and ensure the overall strategy alignment (Exp. 9). Remarkably, one manager mentions his desire to be able to talk to a partner as an equal, which is difficult in a hierarchical organisation such as a hospital (Exp. 6). Therefore, he is glad that he has a good relationship with his chief physicians, with whom he may discuss possible strategic and operational measures, thus reducing potential mistakes.

In addition to the examples of interaction mentioned above, the hospital managers may constrain the physicians when suggestions regarding the implementation of new services, the purchase of medical equipment or recruiting are not in line with the economic situation or the overall strategy of the hospital. In this context, the communication on a matter-of-fact level is essential in order to legitimise the rejection of the corresponding suggestions. Exp. 9, for example, explains that his supervisory board strengthens his position toward the chief physicians in these sorts of discussions:

> During the course of the last year, I find [the board of directors] increasingly helpful because they strengthen my position toward the chief physicians. (. . .) Then I can argue more easily toward my staff and say: "Guys, (. . .) I understand you very well, but there is a clear target from above."

Similarly, managers seek to foster the transparency of budget figures (Exp. 12). If these are known and well-accepted by the chief physicians, they provide a common basis for the discussion of controversial issues. Decisions regarding the purchase of new medical facilities, for instance, are consensually taken by the CEO and the chief physicians based on these figures (Exp. 4).

Furthermore, the hospital managers use incentives to encourage desirable actions. In this respect, the interviewees deliver conflicting statements. On the one hand, some managers mention the effect of monetary incentives on the physicians' motivation: 'At best you address the physicians' wallets' (Exp. 4). On the other hand, Exp. 10 states that money plays a minor role in this context. Instead, physicians are motivated by the leadership style of the CEO. Correspondingly, if the hospital manager ignores their opinion, shows resistance to their advice or gives ambiguous instructions, they are likely to leave the organisation. A mutual appreciation is thus required. Similarly,

Exp. 7 explains that giving orders against the chief physicians' advice does not make sense. He tries, rather, to convince the chief physicians by conducting conversations, either in groups or one-on-one.

Discussion

The findings mentioned above provide insights into the relationship between management and professionals who represent two distinct groups of actors within the hospital as a professional bureaucracy (Mintzberg, 1980). In the following, the results will be discussed in light of the existing literature.

One of the central results of this study is that, in spite of studies assuming a power shift away from the professionals toward the management (e.g. Scott, 1993), managers seem to perceive the medical profession to be a group of powerful actors within the hospital organisation. This corresponds to findings from the existing literature regarding the distinctive role of the professionals within the professional bureaucracy (e.g. Mintzberg, 1980, 2010; Morgan and Ogbonna, 2008; Fiol et al., 2009). Interestingly, the power of the chief physicians not only manifests vis-à-vis the managers of the hospital, but also with respect to the whole organisation through their influence on its reputation. Some managers make use of this circumstance by publishing benchmarking results of their chief physicians in order to demonstrate the superiority of the hospital's performance. On the one hand, this underlines the task of the managers to cope with the external environment (e.g. Mintzberg, 1980; Reeleder et al., 2006), in this case potential personnel and patients. On the other hand, this gives some indication about the managerial scope of action: instead of merely acting as administrators of resources, managers actively utilise the performance results of the chief physicians as a marketing instrument to promote their hospital, thus, exerting control over the professionals – whose performance is publicly evaluated – as well as on the organisational reputation.

In line with Witman et al. (2011), who emphasise the importance of doctors in management positions, the results of this study show that chief physicians contribute substantially to strategy-making processes based on their expert knowledge about medical developments and internal processes. In fact, the physicians are encouraged to make suggestions regarding strategic decisions (bottom-up) by the hospital managers; the assessment of the feasibility and the final approval, however, remains with the CEO and the board of directors (top-down). Apparently, the chief physicians seem to willingly participate in the strategy-making process. This becomes obvious from several examples forwarded by the interviewees regarding strategic initiatives from professionals. On the one hand, this might indicate the professionals' efforts to influence the hospital organisation and, thus, maintain control and reinforce their professional identity (Berg et al., 2000). On the other hand, this points toward the bureaucratisation of the professionals (Lega and Pietro, 2005), who adopt a managerial way of thinking. Corresponding with this bureaucratisation, figures seem to be accepted as a profound basis for discussions at a matter-of-fact level in the case of disagreements between managers and professionals. However, managers also appear to take a step toward the professional culture by emphasising the advantage of having a medical background in managing positions. This manifests an example of the professionalisation of management (Lega and Pietro, 2005).

Relating these findings to Mintzberg's (1980) configuration of the professional bureaucracy, the professionals in the *operating core* seem to have lost some of their power, which has partly been transferred to the *strategic apex* (see Figure 11.1). However, there appears to be an exchange of power rather than an absolute power shift. The chief physicians, indeed, give up some of their control over the development of their medical department, because the final strategic decisions are taken by the managers in the *strategic apex*. However, in return, they receive power back, because they are highly involved in the strategy-making process. Hence, the shift of power seems to be of a mutual, rather than unidirectional, nature. Moreover, the borders between the *strategic apex* and the *operating core* become blurred due to the emergence of hybrid actors possessing both a medical and management background.

Conclusion

In conclusion, this study provides empirical insights into the perception of the medical profession from the managerial point of view and into the interaction between these two groups of actors within the frame of strategy-making in non-profit hospitals. Depending on the medical expertise of the professional staff, the hospital managers appear to involve the chief physicians in the strategy-making process to a high degree. Owing to the exploratory nature of this study, it gives rise to a number of avenues for future research. Further research on the way in which managers may ensure strategy alignment and on how they manage to implement strategies successfully, taking both ethical and economic concerns into account, is required. Implications for the practice, on the one hand, concern the organisational structure of the hospital. The emerging requirement of a close collaboration between managers and doctors questions the vertical authority structure that separates the management of German hospitals into administrative, medical and nursing directors. On the other hand, implications for the education of hospital managers and chief physicians arise. Since chief physicians are, to a great extent, involved in strategic decision-making, an additional economic educational background or appropriate training would be advantageous. Furthermore, hospital CEOs should be selected taking account of their medical knowledge.

Note

1 Supported by the Jackstädt Foundation, in collaboration with Prof. Dr Maximiliane Wilkesmann (TU Dortmund) and Prof. Dr Maik Lachmann (TU Berlin).

References

Anderson, R.A. and McDaniel, R.R. Jr., 2000. Managing health care organizations: where professionalism meets complexity science. *Health Care Management Review*, 25(1), pp. 83–92.

Bär, S., 2011. *Das Krankenhaus zwischen ökonomischer und medizinischer Vernunft. Krankenhausmanager und ihre Konzepte*. Wiesbaden: Springer.

Bazzoli, G.J., 2004. Two decades of organizational change in health care: what have we learned? *Medical Care Research and Review*, 61(3), pp. 247–331.

Berg, M., Horstman, K., Plass, S. and Van Heusden, M., 2000. Guidelines, professionals and the production of objectivity: standardisation and the professionalism of insurance medicine. *Sociology of Health & Illness*, 22(6), pp. 765–91.

Boonstra, A. and Broekhuis, M., 2010. Barriers to the acceptance of electronic medical records by physicians from systematic review to taxonomy and interventions. *BMC Health Services Research*, 10, p. 231.

Federal Statistical Office, 2015a. *Gesundheitsausgaben*. [online] Available through: <www.destatis.de/DE/ZahlenFakten/GesellschaftStaat/Gesundheit/Gesundheitsausgaben/Gesundheitsausgaben.html;jsessionid=638898068F8475973987EAC95FDF1B18.cae2> [accessed 10 May 2015].

Federal Statistical Office, 2015b. *Krankenhäuser*. [online] Available through: <www.destatis.de/DE/ZahlenFakten/GesellschaftStaat/Gesundheit/Krankenhaeuser/Krankenhaeuser.html> [accessed 10 May 2015].

Fiol, C.M., Pratt, M.G. and O'Connor, E.J., 2009. Managing intractable identity conflicts. *Academy of Management Review*, 34(1), pp. 32–55.

Freidson, E., 2001. *Professionalism. The third logic*. Chicago, IL: University of Chicago Press.

Garelick, A., 2005. The doctor-manager relationship. *Advances in Psychiatric Treatment*, 11(4), pp. 241–50.

Kuhlmann, E., Burau, V., Correia, T., Lewandowski, R., Lionis, C., Noordegraaf, M. and Repullo, J., 2013. 'A manager in the minds of doctors': a comparison of new modes of control in European hospitals. *BMC Health Services Research*, 13, p. 246.

Lega, F. and Pietro, C., 2005. Converging patterns in hospital organization: beyond the professional bureaucracy. *Health Policy*, 74(3), pp. 261–81.

Mayring, P., 2000. Qualitative Content Analysis [28 paragraphs]. *Forum Qualitative Sozialforschung/Forum: Qualitative Social Research*. [online] Available through: <http://nbn-resolving.de/urn:nbn:de:0114-fqs0002204> [accessed 05 May 2015].

Mintzberg, H., 1980. Structure in 5'S: a synthesis of the research on organization design. *Management Science*, 26(3), pp. 322–41.

Mintzberg, H., 2010. *Managen*. Offenbach: GABAL Verlag (Management-Reihe).

Morgan, P.I. and Ogbonna, E., 2008. Subcultural dynamics in transformation: a multi-perspective study of healthcare professionals. *Human Relations*, 61(1), pp. 39–65.

Numerato, D., Salvatore, D. and Fattore, G., 2012. The impact of management on medical professionalism: a review. *Sociology of Health & Illness*, 34(4), pp. 626–44.

Reeleder, D., Goel, V., Singer, P.A. and Martin, D.K., 2006. Leadership and priority setting: the perspective of hospital CEOs. *Health Policy*, 79(1), pp. 24–34.

Rohde, J.J., 1962. *Soziologie des Krankenhauses*. Stuttgart: Enke.

Schreyögg, J., Tiemann, O. and Busse, R., 2006. Cost accounting to determine prices: how well do prices reflect costs in the German DRG-system? *Health Care Management Science*, 9(3), pp. 269–79.

Scott, W.R., 1993. The organization of medical care services: toward an integrated theoretical model. *Medical Care Research and Review*, 50(3), pp. 271–303.

Walter, Z. and Lopez, M.S., 2008. Physician acceptance of information technologies: role of perceived threat to professional autonomy. *Decision Support Systems*, 46(1), pp. 206–15.

Wilkesmann, M., 2009. *Wissenstransfer in Krankenhäusern. Strukturelle und institutionelle Voraussetzungen*. Wiesbaden: VS Verlag für Sozialwissenschaften.

Witman, Y., Smid, G.A.C., Meurs, P.L. and Willems, D.L., 2011. Doctor in the lead: balancing between two worlds. *Organization*, 18(4), pp. 477–95.

Part V

Ethical challenges to healthcare professionalism

12 Akrasia and obedience in medicine

Deferring to authority in a decision you believe to be wrong

Tim Wray, Christopher Yu and Christopher Philbey

'The paradoxical and tragic situation of man is that his conscience is weakest when he needs it most.'

Erich Fromm (1947)

Introduction

We, as humans, like to think we can do the right thing when the time comes. We can stand up and say, 'No, I believe that is wrong and I shall not do it.' However, time and time again, it seems we do not stand up, we do not say this and we do what was asked of us anyway.

Physicians make choices for their patients in healthcare everyday – from when to send someone home or into surgery, to which antibiotic a patient should receive. Many of these choices are decided in the upper echelons: the consultants and registrars who have had years of experience. However, these decisions are often implemented by the junior members of the healthcare team. The father of medicine, Hippocrates, teaches that in medicine 'experience [is] perilous, and decision difficult' (Hippocrates, 1984, p. 206).

What happens when there is a disagreement with our seniors or they have made a mistake in judgement? Why in many of these cases do we execute their plans with which we do not agree? What is the emotional cost to the juniors for doing this? Akrasia is the state of acting and doing things against one's better judgement; situations which seem all too common to those in healthcare. Most doctors can probably recall times when they have disagreed with a particular decision but did not challenge it. This chapter does not focus on the good medical practice aspects of the medical decisions, but on the internal moral disagreement arising from the differences of opinions between those issuing the instructions and guidance and those who are tasked with carrying them out. It also looks at how the moral concern can sometimes jar with the professional attitude expected of a junior physician by their seniors.

Mistakes in medicine are a common but not a new stressor. It has recently become more prominent in a doctor's mind with the increased price of the error, as well as the widespread negative press and finger-pointing it often attracts (Well *et al.*, 1997). Levels of stress among doctors, while higher than the average population, have reportedly remained constant: an average of 26.8 per cent of doctors reporting they are stressed, compared to the 17.8 per cent of the general working population (Mizrahi, 1984). Stress in doctors has been shown to decrease quality of care, increase irritability, further mistakes and lead to mental health conditions (Firth–Cozens and Greenhalgh, 1997; Maslach, Schaufeli and Leiter, 2001; Fahrenkopf *et al.*, 2008; Romani and Ashakar, 2014).

This chapter will give an illustration of when junior doctors in a team disagreed with their senior's decision, but did what was requested anyway. It will then look into the reasons why junior doctors choose to go against what they believe they should do, and the additional pressure it can put on them.

Case example

We introduce a case to illustrate the theme of the chapter, which started us asking about obedience to decisions.

A 64–year–old lady with mid–stage progressive bulbar palsy motor neurone disease (MND) was admitted to hospital with a dislocated jaw. Frontal temporal dementia and mutism, evident in this lady, is associated with this condition and, at this point, she lacked mental capacity (Woolley and Katz, 2008; Liillo *et al.*, 2012). Her swallow was assessed and found to be unsafe, partly due to the jaw dislocation, but also the progression of the MND. During several attempts to relocate her mandible by maxillo–facial surgeons, the lady repeatedly self–dislocated her jaw. During this time, while well, alert and receiving intra–venous fluids, she had received no oral calorific intake for 10 days. The patient had had a previous discussion regarding advanced directives with her General Practitioner and Motor Neurone Specialist Nurse (MNSN) several months prior to admission, during which she had non–verbally indicated that she did not want artificial feeding either by nasogastric (NG) or percutaneous end–oscopic gastrostomy (PEG) feeding tubes when it came to the end stage of the disease. It was felt that, at that time, she had capacity to make such a decision. However, it was the opinion of the physicians and neurologist during the current admission that this patient was not at the end stage of the disease and could have several more years of comfortable life remaining if she could receive nutrition.

A 'best interest' meeting was assembled including the patient's son as advocate, dieticians, nurses, the MNSN and physicians' teams to discuss artificial feeding. During this meeting, although the advanced decision was considered, the final decision was to try further NG or PEG feeding, but if insertion of a feeding tube was unsuccessful, further attempts would not be made.

With this outcome decided, the senior clinician requested that his juniors attempt the NG insertion on the ward. This was done with reservation by the junior doctors as they felt it was against what the patient had previously expressed. During the attempted insertion of the NG, the patient became very distressed and unhappy and pulled at the tube. The procedure was stopped and not reattempted as per the original advanced decision by the patient. It left the junior team with a sense of uncertainty as to whether it was right to have tried to insert the feeding tube as instructed.

A brief pilot questionnaire was undertaken by the authors at their local hospitals following the above case to see if this effect was still present among medical doctors. The questions addressed issues around why they implemented a decision with which they did not agree and how integrated the participants felt within their teams. Over a one-month period, there were 40 responses by junior doctors who felt their seniors had made an incorrect decision but who undertook the task requested by the senior clinician anyway. These results highlight there is a clear problem. The possible reasons why this phenomenon occurs will be discussed below.

Discussion

A brief background

There are many famous psychological studies looking at conformity and obedience; Asch (1955) and Milgram (1963) and lesser-known experiments, such as Hofling *et al.* (1966), were undertaken in the 1950s and 1960s. These experiments were undertaken by psychologists to investigate if people would continue to do or say something that they knew would be wrong or harmful just because an authority figure or group said to. However, there are very few modern versions of this research and those that have been published focus little on the reasons why we continue to go against our better judgement, and the stresses it can have on the individual.

It was, perhaps, Stanley Milgram with his famous experiments in 1961 that first really looked into why people continued to do things which they believed were wrong. He was driven by the defences of those tried at the Nuremberg Trials for war crimes post-Second World War: a multitude of people who were able to commit atrocities because they were following orders, despite the latter violating their deepest moral beliefs. His experiments focused on variations of a standard design. This involved a scientist (the authority figure) who ordered the teacher (the subject of the experiment) to give what the subject believed were increasingly painful electrical shocks to a learner (actually an actor complicit with the experiment) each time the learner answered a question wrongly. In reality though, there were no actual punishments, with the learner separated from the subject and told to give predetermined responses to each shock level. If the subjects expressed that they did not want to continue, they were told by the authority that the experiment needed them to continue and that there would be no lasting harm – despite voltages labelled 'Danger! Severe Shock' and accompanied by screams from the learner. The experiment initially found that a staggering 65 per cent gave the full 450 volts, despite being uncomfortable and all participants expressing a wish to stop at some point (Milgram, 1974). This experiment has been repeated over the years and in different countries and displayed consistent findings, although percentages varied (Mantell, 1971; Shanab and Yahya, 1977, 1978; Miranda *et al.*, 1981; Schurz, 1985; Burger, 2009; Blass, 2012).

Effect of culture

On a grand scale, culture and society will inevitably play a significant role in how we interact in the workplace. The psychologist, Geert Hofstede (1983), developed the power distance index (PDI) as a way of quantifying the extent to which the less powerful members of institutions expect and are willing to accept that power is distributed unequally. The PDI is measured numerically: the lower the score indicating a flatter or more equal hierarchy. The UK scores 35, which represents a relatively flat hierarchy and one would assume an ability to challenge authority. This varies worldwide, with countries such as the Philippines or Malaysia having high PDI scores (94 and 104, respectively). The National Health Service, responsible for providing the majority of health-care in the UK, is a highly multicultural organisation bringing expertise from all over the world. The attitudes toward hierarchy by its staff will surely have an impact on their likelihood to challenge authority. A junior from a country with a high PDI might not feel it in their power to challenge anyone in a higher position. It is possible that PDI scores could also be adapted from a top-down perspective as to how a senior member of a team would react to a subordinate if the senior member is from a country with a different PDI score. How this changes the work environment in which the junior doctors find themselves or if they would find it easier to challenge a senior is beyond the scope of this chapter, but is worth mentioning.

Psychology of obedience

Psychologists might suggest that the very structure of a hierarchical system that we obey stems from what Erich Fromm (1947) described as our 'authoritarian conscience'. This is learnt by having the ideal character (a perfect doctor) projected onto an external authority (the senior clinician). Internalisation of this projected perfect character leads to the unwavering belief of the external person as the personification of the perfect figure, leading to the loss of capacity and rationality to question the authoritarian figure. This heteronomous obedience is a submission, one which implies that the individual's will is relinquished to that of the authoritarian figure or the consultant's judgement. It could be this abdicated conscience that enables the individual to believe they are absolved of any error, as the decision was not the individual's but is that of the senior figure. This was proposed by Milgram as his 'agentic state theory' after some of his research participants said during the experiment that it was the researcher's decision to inflict the pain and so the moral guilt was theirs to carry, despite they themselves being the person in final control with the choice of administering the electrical shock or not. They felt their 'hands were clean' as they had been absolved of any responsibility of the outcomes by becoming only a tool for the researcher (Milgram, 1974).

Fromm (1947) had a different perspective, where he considered that it was not guilt that people felt in these situations, but actually fear of disobeying authoritarian commands: commands instilled in us by parents and the state to be submissive to instructions. Regardless of where the guilt or fear which would result from the moral disobedience originates, Fromm's theory is unlikely to fit everyone. However, there are other reasons why doctors might fail to stand up to their senior when they feel it was needed. As junior doctors are still very much in their early stages, they require senior guidance, feedback and assessments of their skill to allow them to progress. This need for approval could lead them to follow a senior clinician's instructions in hope of a reward, and the opposite could also be true. Working as a junior doctor is known to be a busy and stressful job which can only be carried out with the support of colleagues and co-workers. In others areas, juniors are in competition with other colleagues for training opportunities. By showing disobedience, the individual can be stigmatised or isolated from their supporting peers. Fear of being left alone without sympathetic senior support might well contribute to going against their conscience.

Unquestioning obedience – not always a bad thing

The authors are certainly not saying that all decisions from a senior member must be questioned or explained. There are times when questioning would be detrimental to patient care. In an emergency or resuscitation event, for example, a patient is critically unwell and seconds can matter. In this situation, the junior doctor probably has neither the ability nor the experience to make decisions. In these important situations, the individual will often leave the decision-making to the group and its hierarchy. Knowing when to follow an instruction and when not to is not absolute, but situation–dependent.

Within the workplace

Early experiments by Hofling *et al.* (1966) were composed of a telephone instruction to nurses on a ward from an unknown doctor to administer an excessive dose of a fake new medicine 'Astroten'. In the original study, 95 per cent (n = 21) of nurses would have administered the drug. A flaw in this study was that the nurses were not able to contact anybody for advice and that it was an unknown drug. A subsequent study by Rank and Jacobson (1977) attempted to repeat the experiment taking these flaws into account. They did this by using an excessive dose of Valium and allowed the nurses (n = 18) to contact others. The experiment was terminated if they refused the order on the telephone, they prepared the drug, attempted to recall the doctor or allowed more than 15 minutes to pass without taking any action. This study found very different results to that of Hofling *et al.* (1966). While none of the nurses refused on the phone, only 11 per cent (n = 2 of 18) in Rank and Jacobson's study prepared the drug, compared to 95 per cent in the study of Hofling *et al.* Of the 16 who did not prepare the drug, three tried to contact the senior nurse and 12 attempted to re-contact the doctor. This study highlights several key areas regarding all the nurses accepting the doctor's order, but most wanting to question or refuse when they were unsure about its safety and correctness.

One of the reasons that so many of the nurses did not comply was put down by Rank and Jacobson to their familiarity with normal Valium doses. Patricia Brenner's (1982) 'Stages of Clinical Competency' would suggest that this would vary with the expertise of the nurses. The more junior nurses – who Brenner describes as 'novices' or 'advanced beginners', would have difficulty in disobeying, because at such an early stage they lack the discretionary judgement and experience to deviate from the rules and guidelines with which they are trained to know when these guidelines should not be followed – this in the scenario above being 'the nurse's duty to follow a doctor's prescription'. As the individual becomes more competent, they focus less on the rules and more on their past concrete experiences to judge what they would or should do. Those who are more senior are more likely to be familiar with what would constitute a reasonable dose of Valium, would probably have concern over the excessive dose requested and want to be sure before administering it. It could be that the senior clinician is indeed occasionally wrong. Conversely and probably more likely is that just because the junior feels the decision is wrong, does not mean that it is – after all, the seniors have years of experience, knowledge of when to follow the guidelines and when these would be inappropriate. The difficulty here is for the junior to decide when their senior's decision is wrong.

Seeking allies

Within the nurse–Valium study, Rank and Jacobson (1977) noticed that the uncertain nurses discussed with fellow nurses and often sought clarification as to whether or not to give the drug. With this in mind, it is similarly common among juniors to seek out others when concerned about a situation on the ward with which they are not happy. While they might reflect about it to their peers, this empirically does not often seem to result in enough strengthening of will to directly question their senior about the issue. Instead, they sometimes seek allies, often among nurses who have the same duty of care to the patient, but whose hierarchy runs separate and parallel to that of the doctors. Indeed, in one of the variations of Milgram's original experiment (Milgram, 1974), if the teacher/subject was placed with two peer teachers (who were instructed to refuse to continue the experiment) and asked to administer the high level shocks, only 10 per cent instead of the original 65 per cent proceeded to administer the final shock level. In these, whether by strength of numbers or knowing the subjects were not alone in their conflict of conscience, it allowed them to have the will to stand up to the figure of authority. It is easier for doctors in their teams to approach the senior nurses to bring forward their concerns. The nurses will often then voice their concerns directly to the senior clinician as, by their distinct separate roles in the hospital, they are not as at risk from adverse social repercussions during direct confrontation or ensuring refusal of the contentious management plan. Perhaps it is just the lesson that all doctors learn at some point – you ignore nurses at your own peril. Either way, when nursing allies voice their concern by proxy, it can elicit an explanation or change the decision from the senior, as well as alleviate the moral stress of remaining silent.

Addressing the issue

Challenging the hierarchy

There are many potential reasons why individuals do not challenge senior authority even if they think they might have made an incorrect decision. Both the medical and aviation professions have long been expected to function without fault or error. There is emphasis put on self-awareness of fatigue and stress in the training of both professions. However, research by Sexton, Thomas and Helmreich (2000) showed that it is in the airlines where there is more willingness to openly acknowledge limitations: 74 per cent of pilots stated that they did not think they functioned as well when fatigued, compared to 40 per cent of medical professionals. There has been considerable progress in aviation to create a culture which can effectively report and deal with error, which has sadly not progressed as well in medicine, where pressures still exist to cover up mistakes, overlooking opportunities for improvement (de Leval, 1997; Sexton *et al.*, 2000; Scott, 2009; Hoffman and Kanzaria, 2014). Communication skills are key in a constructive path to challenge senior decisions. From this we can take heed from studies carried out by the airline industry and their development of Crew Resource Management. This has also been used in hospital operating theatres and intensive care units with good results, by having senior clinicians open to input and concerns from juniors. Studies (Sexton *et al.*, 2000) have shown that 95 per cent of pilots and consultant anaesthetists advocated flat hierarchies, as opposed to 55 per cent of consultant surgeons. Over 80 per cent of intensive care staff stated that the open nature of their department made it easier to ask questions when they had concerns or did not understand something (Sexton *et al.*, 2000). Crew Resource Management is a five-step standardised procedure used in challenging authority that consists of an opening, a statement that there is a concern, stating the problem as seen by the one with concern, an offer of a solution and finally, an obtainment of agreement. If this technique were to be taught to trainees across all specialities of medicine, it could give team members the confidence to challenge seniors; however, there would probably be resistance from those who feel their decisions should be acted on and not questioned.

Feedback

After the contentious decision is made or instruction carried out, the individual can wrestle with their moral distress at revealing themselves to such risks. The senior's decision could be medically correct, but the junior doctor might feel it to be incorrect due to their own lack of experience, battling against wanting to champion the patient's safety. The unhappiness which can follow such limbo or a detrimental outcome from not challenging the decision, unless turned into a meaningful learning opportunity can negatively influence the doctor throughout their lives.

Studies around the world looking at medical interns and healthcare students concerning professional dilemmas found that unfair criticism of work, erratic feedback and a perceived lack of self-efficacy in their ability to treat patients were the highest ranked stressors in students (Prins *et al.*, 2007; Rees and Monrouxe, 2011; Monrouxe *et al.*, 2014). A study (Paice *et al.*, 2002) between consultants and their juniors found that consultants who were seen as fallible or not supportive led to junior house officers resenting and reconsidering their careers, as well as a lower self-confidence compared to those who felt their seniors were supportive and offered appraisals.

An open culture is needed where questions about decisions which might not have been right can be raised without blame or an explanation regarding why that approach was chosen can be given. Debriefing of junior physicians on the wards rarely happens and is dependent on the individual attitudes of the senior. While junior doctors might talk among themselves, getting genuine instructive senior feedback can be difficult. Their move from being a protected medical student into the future as a medical doctor complete with decision-making and responsibilities is a big transition. With regard to giving feedback, McKimm (2009) highlights the importance of being sensitive and supportive to the needs arising during periods of change and transition in training. She suggests that the focus for a supervisor should be on the events and stressors that might compromise a junior's competence for a period of time (McKimm, 2009; NHS, 2012). McKimm also suggests opportunities at the beginning or end of a feedback session where the trainee can talk about any personal issues that are causing them distress. This approach gives permission to the junior to bring up concerns that are affecting the interplay between 'work' and 'life' (NHS, 2012)

Junior doctors in the UK are assigned clinical supervisors in their working speciality as part of their training posts and it is these with whom they are suggested to discuss or bring concerns. Through this, the supervisor might be able to explain the senior clinician's rationale for their management plan, educating why it was appropriate, or to escalate the individual's concerns if indeed an error has occurred. This debrief can not only allow a vital release of the individual's stress of wrestling with their conscience, but also provides valuable education concerning the event. However, it might be difficult to bring concerns to these supervisors on occasions, as they involve the supervisor's colleagues. This can add fear that if the problem is escalated, then anonymity will be lost and the social repercussions of directly challenging the decisions may still affect the junior.

Conclusion

It is unlikely that any one of these reasons is the single cause of why doctors follow orders with which they do not agree, but it can be said that the issue is present and common among modern day medical practice. Although it might be a minor decision or an outcome from which no harm comes most of the time, this does not make it an easy work environment with such anxiety and stress. An environment without feedback or justification for decisions can lead to a lack of faith in the ability of the leadership and a breakdown of the medical team if left unresolved. Illogical tasks require an increased mental effort, which can result in emotional exhaustion and a career which began as a significant and meaningful vocation becoming unpleasant and unfulfilling. The emotional responses to this strain create irritability, increased work stress and a propensity to ruminate about work-related problems (Maslach *et al.*, 2001; Semmer *et al.*, 2015).

While the authors of this chapter are not trying to say that all juniors live constantly in a hostile work environment where seniors give unethical, incorrect orders and demand the juniors to carry them out against their consciences, there are occasions, for whatever reason, where juniors have issues with instructions and have very little opportunity of resolving them easily. Certain models, such as the CRM, work in some departments of healthcare, but not in all. The difficulty still remains in attempting to tackle the individuals who need to voice their concerns, as well as how those in the position of seniority respond when their directives are questioned. Changing this attitude could be more of a challenge.

Further study

Many of the issues raised here need not be isolated to junior doctors and can be generalised to any hierarchical organisation, it is just that those of the junior doctor are closer to the authors' thoughts. Most of the studies used in this chapter are several decades old, with little revisiting since their original publication. Few have focused on healthcare and fewer still have looked at physicians. The focus of this study has been on the opinion and mindset of the junior doctor, but it has not looked at the problem from the senior doctor's perspective and whether this also occurs at their level between peers.

References

Asch, S., 1955. Opinions and social pressure. *Scientific American*, 192, pp. 31–5.

Blass, T., 2012. A cross-cultural comparison of studies of obedience using the Milgram paradigm: a review. *Social and Personality Psychology Compass*, 6, pp. 196–205.

Brenner, P., 1982. From novice to expert. *American Journal of Nursing*, 82, pp. 402–7.

Burger, J., 2009. Replicating Milgram: would people still obey today? *American Psychologist*, 64, pp. 1–11.

de Leval, M., 1997. Human factors and surgical outcomes: a Cartesian dream. *The Lancet*, 349, pp. 723–5.

Fahrenkopf, A., Sectish, T.C., Barger, L.K., Sharek, P.J., Lewin, D., Chiang, V.W. et al., 2008. Rates of medication errors among depressed and burnt out residents: prospective cohort study. *British Medical Journal*, 336, pp. 488–91.

Firth-Cozens, J. and Greenhalgh, J., 1997. Doctors' perceptions of the links between stress and lowered clinical care. *Social Science & Medicine*, 44, pp. 1017–22.

Fromm, E., 1947. *Man for himself: an inquiry into the psychology of ethics*. New York: Rhinehart & Company Inc.

Hippocrates, 1984. *Hippocratic writings*. Edited by G. Lloyd and J. Chadwick. London: Penguin Books Ltd; reprint edition.

Hoffman, J. and Kanzaria, H.K., 2014. Intolerance of error and culture of blame drive medical excess. *British Medical Journal*, 349, g5702.

Hofling, C.K., Brotzman, E., Dalrymple, S., Graves, N. and Pierce, C.M., 1966. An experimental study in nurse-physician relationships. *Journal of Nervous & Mental Disease*, 143, pp. 171–80.

Hofstede, G., 1983. The cultural relativity of organizational practices and theories. *Journal of International Business Studies*, 14, Special Issue on Cross-Cultural Management, pp. 75–89.

Liillo, P., Savage, S., Mioshi, E., Kiernan, M.C. and Hodges, J.R., 2012. Amyotrophic lateral sclerosis and frontotemporal dementia: a behavioural and cognitive continuum. *Amyotrophic Lateral Sclerosis*, 13, pp. 102–9.

Mantell, D., 1971. The potential for violence in Germany. *Journal of Social Issues*, 27, pp. 101–12.

Maslach, C., Schaufeli, W. and Leiter, M., 2001. Job burnout. *Annual Review of Psychology*, 52, pp. 397–422.

McKimm, P.J., 2009. Giving effective feedback. *British Journal of Hospital Medicine*, 70, pp. 158–61.

Milgram, S., 1963. Behavioral study of obedience. *Journal of Abnormal and Social Psychology*, 67, pp. 371–8.

Milgram, S., 1974. *Obedience to authority: an experimental view*. The University of Michigan: Harper & Row.

Miranda, F., Caballero, R., Gomez, M. and Zamorano, M., 1981. Obediencia a la autoridad [Obedience to authority]. *Psiquis*, 2, pp. 212–21.

Mizrahi, T., 1984. Managing medical mistakes: ideology, insularity and accountability among internists-in-training. *Social Science & Medicine*, 19, pp. 135–46.

Monrouxe, L., Rees, C., Endacott, R. and Ternan, E., 2014. 'Even now it makes me angry': healthcare students' professionalism dilemma narratives. *Medical Education*, 48, pp. 502–17.

NHS: National Health Service Health Education Central & East London, Health Education North West London, Health Education South London, 2012. *Managing the trainee in difficulty*. [Online] Available through: <www.faculty.londondeanery. ac.uk/e-learning/managing-poor-performance> [accessed 19 March 2015].

Paice, E., Moss, F., Heard, S., Winder, B. and McManus, I.C., 2002. The relationship between pre-registration house officers and their consultants. *Medical Education*, 36, pp. 26–34.

Prins, J.T., Gazendam-Donofrio, S.M., Tubben, B.J., van der Heijden, F.M., van de Wiel, H.B. and Hoekstra-Weebers, J.E., 2007. Burnout in medical residents: a review. *Medical Education*, 41, pp. 788–800.

Rank, S. and Jacobson, C., 1977. Hospital nurses' compliance with medication overdose orders: a failure to replicate. *Journal of Health and Social Behavior*, 18, pp. 188–93.

Rees, C. and Monrouxe, L., 2011. 'A morning since eight of just pure grill': a multischool qualitative study of student abuse. *Academic Medicine*, 86, pp. 1374–82.

Romani, M. and Ashakar, K., 2014. Burnout among physicians. *Libyan Journal of Medicine*, 17, p. 23556.

Schurz, G., 1985. Experimentelle Überprüfung des Zusammenhangs zwischen Persönlichkeitsmerkmalen und der Bereitschaft zum destruktiven Gehorsam gegenüber Autoritäten [Experimental examination of the relationships between personality characteristics and the readiness for destructive obedience toward authority]. *Zeitschrift für Experimentelle und Angewandte Psychologie*, 32, pp. 160–77.

Scott, I., 2009. Errors in clinical reasoning: causes and remedial strategies. *British Medical Journal*, 338, p. b1860.

Semmer, N.K., Jacobshagen, N., Meier, L.L., Elfering, A., Beehr, T.A., Kälin, W. and Tschan, F., 2015. Illegitimate tasks as a source of work stress. *Work and Stress*, 29, pp. 32–56.

Sexton, J., Thomas, E. and Helmreich, R., 2000. Error, stress, and teamwork in medicine and aviation: cross sectional surveys. *British Medical Journal*, 320, pp. 645–749.

Shanab, M. and Yahya, K., 1977. A behavioral study of obedience in children. *Journal of Personality and Social Psychology*, 35, pp. 530–6.

Shanab, M. and Yahya, K., 1978. A cross-cultural study of obedience. *Bulletin of the Psychonomic Society*, 11, pp. 267–9.

Well, T.D., Bolden, R.I., Borrill, C.S., Carter, A.J., Golya, D.A., Hardy, G.E. et al., 1997. Minor psychiatric disorder in NHS trust staff: occupational and gender differences. *British Journal of Psychiatry*, 171, pp. 519–23.

Woolley, S. and Katz, J., 2008. Cognitive and behavioral impairment in amyotrophic lateral sclerosis. *Physical Medicine and Rehabilitation Clinics of North America*, 19, pp. 607–17.

13 Professionalism in public health medicine and policy

The challenge of enhancement

Alex McKeown

Introduction

Given the growing threats to health from age-related and preventable lifestyle-related illness in countries such as the UK, there is a need to move as much healthcare provision as possible 'upstream' to optimise and extend healthy longevity (Wanless, 2002; Marmot *et al.*, 2010). The sense in which I use 'professionalism' here is normative. This is to say that while professionalism may be understood as simply obeying codes of conduct, I will concentrate on professionalism understood as what health practitioners and policies *ought* to do.

Understanding of the causes of disease is growing. In the UK,[1] the greatest threats include obesity, unsustainable consumption choices, social isolation, poverty, unemployment and increasingly sedentary lives (NICE, 2014). Sassi and Hurst (2008), for example, estimate that 35 per cent of deaths and 26 per cent of disability-adjusted life years (DALYs) lost in high-income countries are attributable to four modifiable lifestyle factors: smoking, low fruit and vegetable intake, overweight and obesity, and physical inactivity, excluding the effects of these factors on hypertension and high cholesterol.

These are different from the threats faced in previous eras. However, healthcare provision must respond to the needs of society, which are changing. Hanlon *et al.* (2011) and Davies *et al.* (2014) argue that countries such as the UK are experiencing a 'fifth wave' of public health challenges. In contrast to previous waves, which were characterised by the need for remedial treatment, these challenges are preventable by changes that individuals can make to their lifestyles. If this continues and healthcare provision becomes increasingly preventative, the patient–physician relationship will change correspondingly, as Bostrom and Sandberg (2009, p. 332) explain:

> The current rise of personalized medicine results both from improved diagnostic methods that provide a better picture of the individual patient, and from the availability of a wider range of therapeutic options which make it necessary to select the one that is most suitable for a particular patient . . . These factors are leading to a shift in the physician–patient

relationship, away from paternalism to a relationship characterized by teamwork and a focus on the customer's situation. Preventative and enhancing medicine are often inseparable, and both will likely be promoted by these changes.

Prevention aims to ensure ill-health does not occur, and these changes are likely to make it increasingly normal to receive care while still healthy (Chatterjee, 2004; Bostrom and Sandberg, 2009). As a result, an increasing proportion of healthcare provision will be directed to optimising a healthy lifespan, rather than battling disease after it occurs. The changing nature of public health, therefore, may propagate an era in which enhancement plays a growing role, since the enhancement of normal health and functioning will deliver the goal of preventing illness and postponing death (Juengst, 1997; Scripko, 2010). If so, we should think carefully about enhancement's relation to public health.

Enhancement is often 'contraposed' (Bostrom and Roache, 2008) to therapy, which has historically been a more pressing goal of public health. However, if enhancement has – as it appears to – an implicit role to play in public health, regulatory arrangements should reflect this. It is not usually thought of as incumbent on healthcare professionals to provide enhancements – or, at least, not beyond specialities such as private cosmetic surgery (Kinnunen, 2010) or dentistry (Morley, 1999). However, the argument being laid out entails the conclusion that we cannot assume that the restoration of normality constitutes the necessary boundary of appropriate practice.

If this is correct, and public health should focus increasingly on providing care to people in normal health, the concepts of healthcare professionalism will need to change (Goffette, 2006; Drabiak–Syed, 2011), because the prevailing medical model is 'disease focused' (Bostrom and Sandberg, 2009, p. 332). To the (limited) extent that any therapy/enhancement 'distinction' is reliable for providing a dependable guide to what healthcare professions ought and ought not provide, meeting contemporary public health challenges implies accepting that the normative goals of medicine might include procedures which enhance rather than treat. Consequently, recognition that a commitment to the optimisation of healthy longevity might entail the inclusion of enhancements into standard care has significant consequences for healthcare professions.

Enhancement and public health

Although theoretical definitions of enhancement are numerous, they can be summarised broadly as meaning to go beyond 'normal' health and/or functioning. Understood simply, to enhance means to improve, and there is, therefore, an inescapable conceptual connection between the two (Savulescu, 2006; Harris, 2009). However, as Koch (2010) and Capps, Stirrat and Nielson (2012) note, the concept has acquired some overtly individualistic connotations within bioethical discourse, and concerns have been raised that a growth in enhancement medicine will lead to a proliferation of 'schmoctors' (Parens, 1998) who practise enhancement medicine only for profit. Consequently, there is a growing tendency in the literature to look for an account which considers its public health dimensions as well.

Research into the relation between enhancement and public health is nascent. However, a handful of papers have emerged which discuss aspects of it, such as vaccination (Lin and Allhoff, 2008; Lev, Wilfond and McBride, 2013), cognitive enhancement and justice (Nam, 2015), enhancement and prevention in genetics (Juengst, 1997), liberalism and paternalism (Brownsword, 2012), social policy (Loi, Del Savio and Stupka, 2013), and socioeconomic development (Buchanan, 2008). These address specific features of the debate, but a sustained conceptual and ethical analysis of enhancement and public health per se has not yet been done.

Definitions of enhancement

There is insufficient space to deal with each in detail. However, the following rough taxonomy of accounts provides a summary.

Enhancement as 'normal +'

Enhancement via modulation of physiobiological parameters (Canton, 2004; Bostrom and Roache, 2008; Bess, 2010) either within species-typical boundaries, such as the use of erythropoietin (EPO) (Mignon, 2003; Mayes, 2010) or altitude training (Levine, 2006) to increase blood oxygenation for increased endurance in professional sport; or beyond species-typical boundaries, for example, mind-uploading (Kurzweil, 2005; Goertzel and Ikle, 2012) or indefinitely extended lifespan (De Grey, 2005; Kurzweil and Grossman, 2005).

Enhancement relative to personal norms

The term is understood to denote any form of desired improvement, irrespective of one's starting baseline of health or ability (Scully and Rehmann-Sutter, 2001). It could, for example, be equally applied to the use of spectacles to correct defective vision or the use of cognitive enhancing drugs by individuals of normal intelligence with no 'medical need' (Bostrom and Sandberg, 2009; Sandberg and Savulescu, 2011).

Enhancement as an evaluative or normative concept

According to this view, enhancement is understood to be intrinsically morally praiseworthy,[2] since to enhance health means to improve it and the improvement of health is good (Savulescu, 2006; Harris, 2009). Proponents of this view have argued that we have a duty to engage in enhancement (Savulescu, 2005).

Enhancement as 'beyond therapy'

Enhancement understood as the transgression of the boundaries of medicine and distinct from the therapeutic goal of restoring normality (President's Council on Bioethics (U.S.) and Kass, 2003; Pellegrino, 2004).

Definitions of public health

Due to space constraints, I will draw on a similarly broad overview of this field carried out by Dawson and Verweij (2009). The definitions are: positivist descriptions of the public health infrastructure and what it does or does not happen to provide (Kass, 2001); normative, ethically driven analyses of public health which make claims about what the public health infrastructure should and should not provide (Childress *et al.*, 2002; Gostin, 2010); narrow accounts which delimit public health at agencies directly related to healthcare, excluding systems such as education, town planning or sanitation control (Rothstein, 2002); broad accounts which, by contrast, include socio–political, economic welfare systems which exert a causal influence on public health (Baylis, Kenny and Sherwin, 2008; Jennings, 2009); aggregative accounts according to which public health can be understood as the sum total of the health of all the individuals in a given population (Dawson and Verweij, 2009); and distributive accounts which analyse public health according to how equally health variables are spread across the population and, thus, take explicit account of health disparities (Beauchamp, 1980).

The approach to public health that one favours will influence what kind of policies or interventions one believes ought to be provided and accessible. Therefore, opinions differ. Crucially, however, each account shares a common conceptual core, which is adherence to the claim that public health aims at optimising health and ability for the entire population. As Coggon (2012) writes, 'Public health aims its policies toward the community and it counts its results in improved health and longevity in the population.'

With this in mind, to the extent that this statement represents a goal that can be agreed upon beyond differences over other definitional aspects of public health, appropriate policies would be those which successfully deliver this goal. I argue that if improving health and longevity is the goal of public health policy, enhancement cannot be disaggregated from strategies for delivering it. This is not to say that the state should necessarily invest in, for example, radical genetic engineering or providing cognitive enhancing drugs to all. It just indicates that enhancement is *uncontroversially* a goal of public health, and what counts as an appropriate professional response is dynamic, relative to whatever the extant public health challenges happen to be.

Examples of public health enhancement

Many public health successes can be construed as enhancements, for example:

1 *Life expectancy*: normal life expectancy has doubled in the last 200 years (Riley, 2001).
2 *Literacy*: increased cognitive capabilities through education (Freudenberg and Ruglis, 2007).
3 *Child mortality*: this has fallen in Germany from 500 to two per thousand live births in 150 years.[3]
4 *Reduction of infectious diseases* via methods such as effective sanitation (Cutler and Miller, 2005).

These lie within the purview of professional healthcare practice because of the scale of the benefit that they offer. They meet the threshold of acceptability because they are valuable across the whole population, irrespective of relative health or ability. If this is so, we might ask whether other forms of enhancement could do the same, given different public health challenges.

The enhancement debate is frequently discussed in terms of radical and hi-tech interventions, such as genetic engineering (Holtug, 1999; Mehlman, 2005; Rommetveit, 2011) or the use of pharmaceutical products such as Modafinil or Adderall (Greely *et al.*, 2008; Sahakian and Morein-Zamir, 2010; Tannenbaum, 2014). This is misleading, however, because it presents an overly narrow picture of enhancement which, considered more broadly, is less alien than it appears. Effective health enhancement can be achieved using more familiar strategies, for example, regular exercise (Broman-Fulks *et al.*, 2004; De Moor *et al.*, 2006), sustainable consumption choices (Sassi *et al.*, 2009) and political investment in reducing social determinants of ill-health (Harper and Price, 2011). Investment in the sustainable enhancement of public health is needed for the lives people already have, and it is this which constitutes appropriately professional behaviour on behalf of healthcare providers.

Enhancement and therapy

Pursuing this characterisation of enhancement as a familiar phenomenon, it is worth saying something about the putative distinction between therapy and enhancement. The distinction is logically troublesome, because a condition of a therapy's effectiveness is that it enhances. As Pellegrino (2004) notes, there is 'no question that the cure or amelioration of a disease process will also result secondarily in enhancement of the patient's life'.

If this is so, the distinction between prevention and enhancement in the context of public health is even *less* clear, because here we intervene to *extend* health and ability rather than restore it: measures are put in place for sustaining people in normal health, rather than after the onset of illness. Indeed, we can go one step further to say that the concept of enhancement is so pervasive that it is *banal*. On its own, without further circumstantial qualifications about when it is appropriate, the concept of 'enhancement' is bleached of normative content, since all health technologies are instrumentally valuable to the extent that they aim at 'enhancement' via the conferral of an improvement or benefit (Zwart, 2009; Pols and Houkes, 2010).

It is not that these distinctions are completely useless, since they may be heuristically valuable for roughly categorising health needs in order of severity (McKeown, 2014) or for providing an approximate way of distinguishing between those interventions that states should deem it obligatory and non-obligatory to provide (Daniels, 2000). However, appropriate professional practice must be driven by a commitment to the hierarchy of needs that the therapy/enhancement distinction implies, rather than where precisely on that hierarchy the distinction is made. Health needs change as society changes, and what constitutes appropriate professional practice must be recognised as needing to be similarly dynamic, as Savulescu (2006) has argued:

> [W]hat IQ is necessary for a decent chance of a decent life? Perhaps, in a technologically sophisticated society, people would significantly benefit from a higher IQ. An IQ of 120 is needed to be able to complete tertiary education . . . justice requires enhancement. It is on these grounds that we choose to treat those currently with an IQ less than 70. But where we set the minimum threshold for treatment or enhancement is up to us.

Case study: enhancement and the normal haematocrit

As an illustration, I will draw on an empirical study[4] carried out as part of a PhD project investigating the therapy/enhancement distinction (McKeown, 2014). The aims were:

1   to understand how therapy/enhancement distinction is viewed within medicine;
2   to understand the ethical concerns associated with these views;
3   to identify justifications informing these views in order to carry out an analysis of them;
4   to give a refined account of therapy/enhancement informed by both theory and data.

It was necessary to identify an appropriate case study which could yield relevant data. Synthetic recombinant erythropoietin (EPO) was chosen. This is a widely used pharmaceutical developed for therapeutic purposes, but which is also used for enhancement (Fisher, 2010; Mayes, 2010).

EPO is a copy of the hormone erythropoietin produced by the kidneys which stimulates red blood cell production in the bone-marrow. Red cells contain haemoglobin, and erythropoietin is, thus, implicated in ensuring adequate oxygen supply (Jelkmann, 2007). It is administered when kidney function declines, since when this occurs, erythropoietin production decreases, the red cell count falls and the individual develops anaemia, becoming progressively more lethargic and fatigued and, left untreated, it results in death (MacDougall *et al.*, 1990). EPO mimics endogenous erythropoietin by maintaining red cell production and, thus, ensuring an adequate oxygen supply, or 'haematocrit', which reverses the symptoms of anaemia (Wenger and Kurtz, 2011).

EPO was introduced into clinical practice in the late-1980s (MacDougall *et al.*, 1990; Winearls, 2006), and since it is both effective at boosting physical performance and hard to detect, it was rapidly appropriated for clandestine enhancement use in sport, most notably in professional cycling (Mignon, 2003; Diamanti-Kandarakis *et al.*, 2005; Robinson, 2006). EPO mimics the effects of legal methods of increasing blood oxygenation, such as altitude training or the use of hypoxic chambers (Joyner, 2003), and has been implicated in high-profile 'doping' cases, such as those of Lance Armstrong and David Millar.[5]

Having identified the case study, relevant participants were contacted for interview. These were clinical nephrologists and renal scientists, 25 of whom were interviewed. All were drawn from the National Health Service, but answered in an 'independent' capacity. The interviews were an epistemological, ontological and ethical investigation into the views that they held about the concept of human enhancement and its relation to therapy, for example:

1 questions about the logical reducibility of therapy to enhancement;
2 whether they had good reasons for distinguishing between therapy and enhancement;
3 whether there are good arguments to exclude enhancement from standard medical practice.

The study yielded a wealth of data, so I will focus on one aspect of particular relevance to the present purpose which relates to the adequacy of a species-typical haematocrit.

A standard human haematocrit ranges from 13–17 g/dl (Lacson, Ofsthun and Lazarus, 2003). EPO is typically administered once the haematocrit falls beneath 10 g/dl, as this is the threshold at which symptoms of anaemia tend to occur (Will, 2001; Will *et al.*, 2007). One might think that the appropriate therapeutic strategy would be to restore the haematocrit to within the species-typical 13–17 g/dl range (Paoletti and Cannella, 2006; Szczech *et al.*, 2008). However, this is not the case. Typically, the therapeutic benefit begins to tail off the further above 10 g/dl that one moves (Singh *et al.*, 2006; Besarab *et al.*, 2012) and the concomitant risk of thrombosis increases from the thickening of the blood caused by extra red blood cells (Remuzzi and Ingelfinger, 2006; Fishbane and Wish, 2012). The reasons for this are not fully understood (Fishbane and Wish, 2012). It could be, for example, because EPO is not a perfect copy of the endogenous molecule and the body has an adverse reaction to it for reasons that are currently unknown (Fishbane, 2009). Alternatively, undiscovered erythro-poietin receptors might exist elsewhere in the body alongside the bone-marrow receptors (Winter *et al.*, 2005) which are the target of EPO replacement therapy. These, in addition to the bone-marrow receptors, may detect the presence of EPO when it is injected, causing an unanticipated spike in red cell production which thickens the blood, raising the risk of thrombosis.

One hypothesis suggested, however, was that a species-typical haematocrit is higher than necessary for the demands of twenty-first century living. Current threats to health in a country such as the UK are different from those of the evolutionary environment in which humans emerged (Warnock, 2003; Powell and Buchanan, 2011). For example, we do not have to hunt for food or fear starvation, we are not preyed on by wild animals that we need to out-run, less blood is lost in childbirth, and so on. Contemporary life is less harsh than in that environment and it is at least possible that we now have more haemoglobin than we need, as daily threats that would have required a greater capacity for physical endurance to resist have receded.

If this hypothesis is correct, it follows that we may be at an unnecessarily high risk of thrombosis, relative to other threats to life. Although the risk may be negligible, nevertheless, it gives credence to the claim that we may be maladapted because the balance between our biology and our environment has changed. This conclusion is redolent of arguments made by Bostrom and Sandberg (2009) about the 'moving target' (Bess, 2010) of enhancement. Bostrom and Sandberg (2009, p. 381) summarise the radical difference between the 'environment of evolutionary adaptedness' (EEA) and the present day by pointing out that '[h]unting, gathering of fruits and nuts, courtship, parasites, and hand-to-hand combat with wild animals and enemy tribes were elements of the EEA; speeding cars, high levels of trans fats, concrete ghettos, and tax return forms were not.'

In our case, having a haematocrit that is marginally higher than necessary is not a serious enough risk to health to warrant its systematic reduction in the name of public health, but the case is illustrative. Again, identifying public health priorities – in other words, those that are writ large across the whole population – means identifying risk factors common not just to disease communities. Having done so, professional behaviour consists of making a judgement about the importance of these relative to other needs and finding ways to mitigate them by optimising those characteristics if needed.

Professionalism, enhancement and public health

In the present day, if improved public health succeeds in moving care 'upstream' away from remediation toward prevention, an appropriately professional policy response would seek to extend healthy lifespans and optimise our decision-making capabilities with respect to the achievement of this goal.

However, this still leaves open the question of what technologies or interventions should be used to achieve it. It may be, as Bostrom (2004) and More and Vita-More (2013) have argued, that cutting-edge biotechnological solutions, such as genetic neuroenhancement (Savulescu, 2005; Sandberg, 2011) and biogerontology (De Grey, 2005, 2007), can best deliver the goals of improved cognition and extended healthy lifespan required.

Alternatively, however, less hi-tech interventions, such as increased exercise or better education, may be preferable for morally significant reasons. These could include the holistic value of exercise for both mental and physical health (Taylor *et al.*, 1985; Fox, 1999; Paluska and Schwenk, 2000) and the cultivation of sociability that schooling enables beyond academic learning (McMahon, 2004; Schuller *et al.*, 2004). Although both access to and the quality of education are unequal, in countries such as the UK it is, nevertheless, provided freely to all children by the state. Similarly, exercise, while sometimes requiring financial commitment, can in general be engaged in cheaply. Consequently, lo-tech interventions such as these are *prima facie* favourable in the present, since they are at least accessible to all and not just the rich. If these are preferable to biotechnological solutions, it is they that healthcare professions should implement.

Of course, just because this conclusion is acceptable *in the present* does not mean that it will be in the future, since our needs and the threats to life might change. When looking to the future, the post-humanist arm of enhancement philosophy (Bostrom, 2005; Kurzweil, 2005; More and Vita-More, 2013) becomes relevant. Were our circumstances to change significantly, what counts as an appropriately professional public health response would also change according to the occurrence of new risks. The field of existential risk studies (Matheny, 2007), for example, has identified potentially imminent threats to the survival of the human race, such as catastrophic man-made environmental damage (Thomas *et al.*, 2004; Bostrom, 2013) or the emergence of a machine-based superintelligence which decides that it is in its interests to terminate human existence (Yudkowsky, 2008; Bostrom, 2014).

These might appear to be far-fetched 'sci-fi' possibilities. However, even if the risks are remote or distant, they illustrate that in certain emergency scenarios it could be necessary for the human race to alter itself dramatically in order to survive, and in doing so, bring about a post-human – in other words, human atypical – era (Schneider, 2009; Bishop, 2010). Even if the scenarios outlined here *never* occur, the thought experiment raises a significant point about public health. Irrespective of the situation we find ourselves in now, what may be considered a responsible, professional or appropriate public health response is dynamic and might go far beyond our present norms.

Conclusions

In concluding, we should ask what would count as an appropriately professional approach to enhancement in public health medicine and policy. The answer is unremarkable, since the conditions of professionalism remain the same irrespective of whatever intervention or policy is under consideration. In a public health context, professional behaviour is grounded in providing those interventions that are most cost-effective in successfully optimising healthy longevity across a population in a way that does not exacerbate disparities in accessing the benefits of those interventions.

Furthermore, it is a condition of any effective health intervention that it enhances, regardless of whether it is administered to somebody ill or somebody healthy. Although there are qualitative differences between health interventions to the extent that they are effective, the conceptual association with enhancement persists. This is true even if enhancement in the sense of achieving a state of radical supra–normality is not the reason for intervening. It is possible, for example, to aim at optimising or extending healthy longevity because one judges that it is bad to become ill, and make no reference to enhancement. Nevertheless, if a healthy lifespan is successfully optimised or extended, the intervention will have conferred an enhancement, even if this is just a side–effect.

Threats to public health are not static, and what is required to meet changing threats must be similarly dynamic. In the UK and other developed nations, for example, the threat of death from infectious disease has diminished dramatically, but there has been a significant increase in death from unsustainable lifestyle choices. Preventing death from such choices consists of being able to create situations in which the public can both take responsibility for its own health and receive ongoing assistance while healthy to extend that state as long as possible. As a result, the particular challenges faced in countries such as the UK may increasingly entail the need to enhance the lifespan of an already healthy population.

The difficulty in making the case for enhancement understood as a necessary and unremarkable feature of public health provision follows, in part, from the individualistic, neo–liberal flavour that has come to be associated with the term. This is changing, however, and increasingly there is evidence within the enhancement discourse of a recognition that enhancement may be a more banal issue than has been presented, at least with respect to the parochial, incremental context of public policy–making. Public health is already concerned with enhancement, since the aim is to improve lives through better health.

It is true that the further we look into the future, the more speculative the risk scenarios become. Nevertheless, if they were to occur, a professional response from the healthcare professions would consist of mitigating those risks, whatever they happened to be. Despite the apparent transcendence of enhancement beyond the boundary of medical and healthcare practice, we cannot guarantee that those boundaries will remain static. Public health needs will continue to change and it is a recognition of this which can orientate an appropriately professional attitude to policy development.

Acknowledgements

This work was funded by a Wellcome Trust Society and Ethics Small Grant under the project 'Ethics, Enhancement and Public Health'. Thanks to the Wellcome Trust for their support.

Notes

1 Different countries may well have correspondingly different healthcare systems and infrastructures, however, there is insufficient space to explore this. My research relates to the UK context and I, therefore, acknowledge potential limitations of my conclusions.
2 It is fair to note that this account has been met with scepticism. Shickle (2000) Fukuyama (2002), Habermas (2003), President's Council on Bioethics (U.S.) and Kass (2003), Sandel (2004), and Koch (2010), among others, have expressed concerns. Their arguments contend that (a) enhancement will be inevitably unjust because we live in a market-orientated world, and since access to enhancements will be determined by wealth, it is probable that the benefits will accrue to the rich, thus, exacerbating existing socioeconomic injustices; (b) enhancements are undesirable because they devalue the adequacy of normal health and functioning, and will be inherently coercive, as people will feel that they must enhance if they wish to 'keep up' in society; (c) enhancement is pernicious because it is eugenicism 'cloaked' in a guise of autonomy and self-determination which will not protect people from injustices because of the societal impacts of (a) and (b); and (d) it cannot be inferred from the fact that something 'enhances' that it is necessarily good. For example, I could 'enhance' my chances of killing somebody with a gun rather than my hands, but it does not follow that this is ethically desirable. There are other arguments, but these are the most significant, and space forbids a fuller exposition here.
3 <http://ourworldindata.org/data/population-growth-vital-statistics/life-expectancy/> [accessed on 16 October 2015].
4 Permission granted by the University of Bristol Faculty of Medicine and Dentistry Committee for Ethics on 20 December 2011, ref: 111208.
5 <www.bbc.co.uk/news/world-europe-20026838>; <http://news.bbc.co.uk/1/hi/programmes/hardtalk/9571648.stm> [accessed on 16 October 2015].

References

Baylis, F., Kenny, N.P. and Sherwin, S., 2008. A relational account of public health ethics. *Public Health Ethics*, 1, pp. 196–209.

Beauchamp, D.E., 1980. Public health and individual liberty. *Annual Review of Public Health*, 1, pp. 121–36.

Besarab, A., Kline Bolton, W.K., Nissenson, A.R. and Schwab, S.J., 2012. The normal HCT trial re-revisited: what were the actual findings? *Kidney International*, 82, p. 242.

Bess, M., 2010. Enhanced humans versus 'normal people': elusive definitions. *Journal of Medicine and Philosophy*, 35, pp. 641–55.

Bishop, J.P., 2010. Transhumanism, metaphysics, and the posthuman god. *Journal of Medicine and Philosophy*, 35, pp. 700–20.

Bostrom, N., 2004. The future of human evolution. In: C. Tandy ed., *Death and anti-death: two hundred years after Kant, fifty years after Turing*. Palo Alto, CA: Ria University Press. pp. 339–71.

Bostrom, N., 2005. A history of transhumanist thought. *Journal of Evolution and Technology*, 14(1), pp. 1–25.

Bostrom, N., 2013. Existential risk prevention as global priority. *Global Policy*, 4, pp. 15–31.

Bostrom, N., 2014. *Superintelligence: paths, dangers, strategies*. Oxford: Oxford University Press.

Bostrom, N. and Roache, R., 2008. Ethical issues in human enhancement. In: J. Ryberg, T. Petersen and C. Wolf eds., *New waves in applied ethics*. London: Palgrave Macmillan, pp. 120–52.

Bostrom, N. and Sandberg, A., 2009. Cognitive enhancement: methods, ethics, regulatory challenges. *Science and Engineering Ethics*, 15, pp. 311–41.

Broman-Fulks, J.J., Berman, M.E., Rabian, B.A. and Webster, M.J., 2004. Effects of aerobic exercise on anxiety sensitivity. *Behaviour Research and Therapy*, 42, pp. 125–36.

Brownsword, R., 2012. Five principles for the regulation of human enhancement. *Asian Bioethics Review*, 4, pp. 344–54.

Buchanan, A., 2008. Enhancement and the ethics of development. *Kennedy Institute of Ethics Journal*, 18, pp. 1–34.

Canton, J., 2004. Designing the future: NBIC technologies and human performance enhancement. *Annals of the New York Academy of Sciences*, 1013, pp. 186–98.

Capps, B.J., Stirrat, G. and Nielson, L.W., 2012. A brief critique of two claims about the social value of biotechnological enhancements. *Asian Bioethics Review*, 4, pp. 259–71.

Chatterjee, A., 2004. Cosmetic neurology: the controversy over enhancing movement, mentation, and mood. *Neurology*, 63, pp. 968–74.

Childress, J.F., Faden, R.R., Gaare, R.D., Gostin, L.O., Kahn, J., Bonnie, R.J. *et al.*, 2002. Public health ethics: mapping the terrain. *Journal of Law, Medicine & Ethics*, 30, pp. 170–8.

Coggon, J., 2012. *What makes health public? A critical evaluation of moral, legal, and political claims in public health.* Cambridge, UK: Cambridge University Press.

Cutler, D. and Miller, G., 2005. The role of public health improvements in health advances: the twentieth-century United States. *Demography*, 42, pp. 1–22.

Daniels, N., 2000. Normal functioning and the treatment-enhancement distinction. *Cambridge Quarterly of Healthcare Ethics*, 9, pp. 309–22.

Davies, S.C., Winpenny, E., Ball, S., Fowler, T., Rubin, J. and Nolte, E., 2014. For debate: a new wave in public health improvement. *The Lancet*, 384, pp. 1889–95.

Dawson, A. and Verweij, M., 2009. *Ethics, prevention, and public health.* Oxford, UK: Oxford University Press.

De Grey, A.D.N.J., 2005. Life extension, human rights, and the rational refinement of repugnance. *Journal of Medical Ethics*, 31, pp. 659–63.

De Grey, A.D.N.J., 2007. Life span extension research and public debate: societal considerations. *Studies in Ethics, Law and Technology*, 1, p. 5.

De Moor, M.H.M., Beem, A.L., Stubbe, J.H., Boomsma, D.I. and De Geus, E.J.C., 2006. Regular exercise, anxiety, depression and personality: a population-based study. *Preventive Medicine*, 42, pp. 273–9.

Diamanti-Kandarakis, E., Konstantinopoulos, P.A., Papailiou, J., Kandarakis, S.A., Andreopoulos, A. and Sykiotis, G.P., 2005. Erythropoietin abuse and erythropoietin gene doping. *Sports Medicine*, 35, pp. 831–40.

Drabiak-Syed, K., 2011. Physicians prescribing 'medicine' for enhancement: why we should not and cannot overlook safety concerns. *American Journal of Bioethics*, 11, pp. 17–19.

Fishbane, S., 2009. Erythropoiesis-stimulating agent treatment with full anemia correction: a new perspective. *Kidney International*, 75, pp. 358–65.

Fishbane, S. and Wish, J.B., 2012. A physician's perseverance uncovers problems in a key nephrology study. *Kidney International*, 82, pp. 135–7.

Fisher, J.W., 2010. Landmark advances in the development of erythropoietin. *Experimental Biology and Medicine*, 235, pp. 1398–411.

Fox, K.R., 1999. The influence of physical activity on mental well-being. *Public Health Nutrition*, 2, pp. 411–18.

Freudenberg, N. and Ruglis, J., 2007. Peer reviewed: reframing school dropout as a public health issue. *Preventing Chronic Disease*, 4, p. A107.

Fukuyama, F., 2002. *Our posthuman future.* New York: Saint Martin's Press Inc.

Goertzel, B. and Ikle, M., 2012. Mind uploading (introduction to a special issue on this topic). *International Journal of Machine Consciousness*, 4, pp. 1–3.

Goffette, J., 2006. *Naissance de l'anthropotechnie: de la médecine au modelage de l'humain.* Paris, France: Librarie Philosophique J. Vrin.

Gostin, L.O. ed., 2010. *Public health law and ethics: a reader.* Vol. 4. Oakland, CA: University of California Press.

Greely, H., Sahakian, B., Harris, J., Kessler, R.C., Gazzaniga, M., Campbell, P. and Farah, M.J., 2008. Towards responsible use of cognitive-enhancing drugs by the healthy. *Nature*, 456, pp. 702–5.

Habermas, J., 2003. *The future of human nature.* Hoboken, NJ: John Wiley & Sons.

Hanlon, P., Carlisle, S., Hannah, M., Reilly, D. and Lyon, A., 2011. Making the case for a 'fifth wave' in public health. *Public Health*, 125, pp. 30–36.

Harper, G. and Price, R., 2011. *A framework for understanding the social impacts of policy and their effects on wellbeing.* London: Department for Environment, Food, and Rural Affairs.

Harris, J., 2009. Enhancements are a moral obligation. In: N. Bostrom, and J. Savulescu eds., *Human enhancement.* Oxford: Oxford University Press, pp. 131–54.

Holtug, N., 1999. Does justice require genetic enhancements? *Journal of Medical Ethics*, 25, pp. 137–43.

Jelkmann, W., 2007. Erythropoietin after a century of research: younger than ever. *European Journal of Haematology*, 78, pp. 183–205.

Jennings, B., 2009. Public health and liberty: beyond the Millian paradigm. *Public Health Ethics*, 2, pp. 123–34.

Joyner, M.J., 2003. O_2MAX, blood doping, and erythropoietin. *British Journal of Sports Medicine*, 37, pp. 190–1.

Juengst, E.T., 1997. Can enhancement be distinguished from prevention in genetic medicine? *Journal of Medicine and Philosophy*, 22, pp. 125–42.

Kass, N.E., 2001. An ethics framework for public health. *American Journal of Public Health*, 91, pp. 1776–82.

Kinnunen, T., 2010. 'A second youth': pursuing happiness and respectability through cosmetic surgery in Finland. *Sociology of Health & Illness*, 32, pp. 258–71.

Koch, T., 2010. Enhancing who? Enhancing what? Ethics, bioethics, and transhumanism. *Journal of Medicine and Philosophy*, 35, pp. 685–99.

Kurzweil, R., 2005. *The singularity is near: when humans transcend biology.* New York: Viking Penguin.

Kurzweil, R. and Grossman, T., 2005. *Fantastic voyage: live long enough to live forever.* New York: Rodale.

Lacson, E., Ofsthun, N. and Lazarus, M.J., 2003. Effect of variability in anemia management on hemoglobin outcomes in ESRD. *American Journal of Kidney Diseases*, 41, pp. 111–24.

Lev, O., Wilfond, B.S. and McBride, C.M. (2013). Enhancing children against unhealthy behaviors – an ethical and policy assessment of using a nicotine vaccine. *Public Health Ethics*, pht006.

Levine, B.D., 2006. Should 'artificial' high altitude environments be considered doping? *Scandinavian Journal of Medicine and Science in Sports*, 16, pp. 297–301.

Lin, P. and Allhoff, F., 2008. Untangling the debate: the ethics of human enhancement. *NanoEthics*, 2, pp. 251–64.

Loi, M., Del Savio, L. and Stupka, E., 2013. Social epigenetics and equality of opportunity. *Public Health Ethics*, 6, pp. 142–53.

MacDougall, I.C., Hutton, R.D., Cavill, I., Coles, G.A. and Williams, J.D., 1990. Treating renal anaemia with recombinant human erythropoietin: practical guidelines and a clinical algorithm. *British Medical Journal*, 300, p. 655.

Marmot, M.G., Allen, J., Goldblatt, P., Boyce, T., McNeish, D., Grady, M. and Geddes, I., 2010. *Fair society, healthy lives: strategic review of health inequalities in England post-2010*. London, UK: The Marmot Review.

Matheny, J.G., 2007. Reducing the risk of human extinction. *Risk Analysis*, 27, pp. 1335–44.

Mayes, R., 2010. The modern Olympics and post-modern athletics: a clash in values. *The Journal of Philosophy, Science & Law*, 10, pp. 1–17.

McKeown, A., 2014. *Re-thinking the distinction between therapy and enhancement: a study in empirical ethics*. Unpublished thesis. University of Bristol.

McMahon, W.W., 2004. The social and externality benefits of education. In: G. Johnes and J. Johnes eds., *International handbook on the economics of education*. Cheltenham, UK: Edward Elgar Publications, pp. 211–59.

Mehlman, M.J., 2005. Genetic enhancement: plan now to act later. *Kennedy Institute of Ethics Journal*, 15, pp. 77–82.

Mignon, P., 2003. The Tour de France and the doping issue. *International Journal of the History of Sport*, 20, pp. 227–45.

More, M. and Vita-More, N. eds., 2013. *The transhumanist reader: classical and contemporary essays on the science, technology, and philosophy of the human future*. Hoboken, NJ: John Wiley & Sons.

Morley, J., 1999. The role of cosmetic dentistry in restoring a youthful appearance. *Journal of the American Dental Association*, 130, pp. 1166–72.

Nam, J., 2015. Biomedical enhancements as justice. *Bioethics*, 29, pp. 126–32.

NICE: National Institute of Clinical Excellence, Local Government Briefings, 2014. *Community engagement to improve health*. London, UK: National Institute of Clinical Excellence.

Paluska, S.A. and Schwenk, T.L., 2000. Physical activity and mental health. *Sports Medicine*, 29, pp. 167–80.

Paoletti, E. and Cannella, G., 2006. Update on erythropoietin treatment: should hemoglobin be normalized in patients with chronic kidney disease? *Journal of the American Society of Nephrology*, 17, pp. S74–S77.

Parens, E., 1998. Is better always good? The enhancement project. *Hastings Center Report*, 28, pp. s1–s17.

Pellegrino, E., 2004. Biotechnology, human enhancement, and the ends of medicine. *The Center for Bioethics & Human Dignity*, [online]. Available through: <https://cbhd.org/content/biotechnology-human-enhancement-and-ends-medicine> [accessed 11 September 2015].

Pols, A.J.K. and Houkes, W., 2010. What is morally salient about enhancement technologies? *Journal of Medical Ethics*, 37, pp. 84–7.

Powell, R. and Buchanan, A., 2011. Breaking evolution's chains: the prospect of deliberate genetic modification in humans. *Journal of Medicine and Philosophy*, 36, pp. 6–27.

President's Council on Bioethics (U.S.) and Kass, L., 2003. *Beyond therapy: biotechnology and the pursuit of happiness*. New York: Regan Books.

Remuzzi, G. and Ingelfinger, J.R., 2006. Correction of anemia-payoffs and problems. *New England Journal of Medicine*, 355, p. 2144.

Riley, J.C., 2001. *Rising life expectancy: a global history*. Cambridge, UK: Cambridge University Press.

Robinson, N., 2006. Erythropoietin and blood doping. *British Journal of Sports Medicine*, 40, pp. i30–i34.

Rommetveit, K., 2011. Genetic enhancement, futures tense. *Futures*, 43, pp. 76–85.

Rothstein, M.A., 2002. Rethinking the meaning of public health. *Journal of Law, Medicine & Ethics*, 30, pp. 144–9.

Sahakian, B.J. and Morein-Zamir, S., 2010. Neuroethical issues in cognitive enhancement. *Journal of Psychopharmacology*, 25, pp. 197–204.

Sandberg, A., 2011. Cognition enhancement: upgrading the brain. In: J. Savulescu, R. Ter Meulen and G. Kahane eds., *Enhancing human capacities*. Oxford, UK: Wiley-Blackwell, pp. 71–91.

Sandberg, A. and Savulescu, J., 2011. The social and economic impacts of cognitive enhancement. In: J. Savulescu, R. Ter Meulen and G. Kahane eds., *Enhancing human capacities*. Oxford, UK: Wiley-Blackwell, pp. 92–112.

Sandel, M., 2004. The case against perfection. *Atlantic Monthly*, 293, pp. 51–62.

Sassi, F. and Hurst, J. 2008. The prevention of lifestyle-related chronic diseases: an economic framework. [online]. Available through <www.oecd.org/els/health-systems/40324263.pdf> [accessed 12 February 2016].

Sassi, F., Cecchini, M., Lauer, J. and Chisholm, D., 2009. *Improving lifestyles, tackling obesity: the health and economic impact of prevention strategies (No. 48)*. Paris, France: OECD Publishing.

Savulescu, J., 2005. New breeds of humans: the moral obligation to enhance. *Reproductive BioMedicine Online*, 10, pp. 36–9.

Savulescu, J., 2006. Justice, fairness, and enhancement. *Annals of the New York Academy of Sciences*, 1093, pp. 321–38.

Schneider, S., 2009. Mindscan: transcending and enhancing the human brain. In: S. Schneider ed., *Science fiction and philosophy: from time travel to superintelligence*. Chichester, UK: Wiley, pp. 241–56.

Schuller, T., Hammond, C., Preson, J., Brassett-Grundy, A. and Bynner, J., 2004. *The benefits of learning: the impact of education on health, family life and social capital*. London, UK: Routledge.

Scripko, P.D., 2010. Enhancement's place in medicine. *Journal of Medical Ethics*, 36, pp. 293–6.

Scully, J.L. and Rehmann-Sutter, C., 2001. When norms normalize: the case of genetic 'enhancement'. *Human Gene Therapy*, 12, pp. 87–95.

Shickle, D., 2000. Are 'genetic enhancements' really enhancements? *Cambridge Quarterly of Healthcare Ethics*, 9, pp. 342–52.

Singh, A.K., Szczech, L., Tang, K.L., Barnhart, H., Sapp, S., Wolfson, M. and Reddan, D., 2006. Correction of anemia with epoetin alfa in chronic kidney disease. *New England Journal of Medicine*, 355, pp. 2085–98.

Szczech, L.A., Barnhart, H.X., Inrig, J.K., Reddam, D.N., Sapp, S., Califf, R.M. et al., 2008. Secondary analysis of the CHOIR trial epoetin-α dose and achieved hemoglobin outcomes. *Kidney International*, 74, pp. 791–8.

Tannenbaum, J., 2014. The promise and peril of the pharmacological enhancer Modafinil. *Bioethics*, 28, pp. 436–45.

Taylor, C., Barr, J., Sallis, F. and Needle, R., 1985. The relation of physical activity and exercise to mental health. *Public Health Reports*, 100, p. 195.

Thomas, C.D., Cameron, A., Green, R.E., Bakkenes, M., Beaumont, L.J., Collingham, Y.C. and Erasmus, F.N.B., 2004. Extinction risk from climate change. *Nature*, 427, pp. 145–8.

Wanless, D., 2002. *Securing our future health: taking a long-term view*. London, UK: HM Treasury.

Warnock, M., 2003. What is natural? And should we care? *Philosophy*, 78, pp. 445–59.

Wenger, R.H. and Kurtz, A., 2011. Erythropoietin. *Comprehensive Physiology*, 1, pp. 1759–94.

Will, E.J. 2001. Aiming at averages. *Journal of the Royal Society of Medicine*, 94(12), pp. 617–19.

Will, E.J., Richardson, D., Tolman, C. and Bartlett, C., 2007. Development and exploitation of a clinical decision support system for the management of renal anaemia. *Nephrology Dialysis Transplantation*, 22, pp. iv31–iv36.

Winearls, C.G., 2006. In the wake of progress: ethical problems of renal failure treated by dialysis. *Clinical Medicine*, 6, pp. 76–80.

Winter, S.C., Shah, K.A., Campo, L., Turley, H., Leek, R., Corbridge, R.J., Cox, G.J. and Harris, A.L., 2005. Relation of erythropoietin and erythropoietin receptor expression to hypoxia and anemia in head and neck squamous cell carcinoma. *Clinical Cancer Research*, 11, pp. 7614–20.

Yudkowsky, E., 2008. Artificial intelligence as a positive and negative factor in global risk. *Global Catastrophic Risks*, 1, p. 303.

Zwart, H., 2009. From Utopia to science: challenges of personalised genomics information for health management and health enhancement. *Medicine Studies*, 1, pp. 155–66.

14 Ethics and professionalism in healthcare

A position paper[1]

More than a decade ago, the powerful statement 'Medical Professionalism in the New Millennium: A Physician Charter' was launched by three medical organisations: the American College of Physicians–American Society of Internal Medicine (ACP-ASIM) Foundation, the American Board of Internal Medicine (ABIM) Foundation and the European Federation of Internal Medicine. It has been endorsed by more than 130 organisations across the world and has been translated into 120 languages (ABIM Foundation, 2015). The Charter expresses an attempt to defend the medical profession's integrity against external factors, such as political, legal and market forces (ABIM Foundation, 2002). Based on the three principles of patient welfare, patient autonomy and social justice, the Charter aims at formulating a contemporary understanding of physicians' status as a profession.

Professionalism in healthcare is evolving rapidly. Societal, legal and medico-technical developments (such as changing compensation systems, increasing sub-specialisation or new medical devices) necessitate constant development regarding the role of physicians and other professions in healthcare. The contributions in this volume are the result of an interdisciplinary conference for young scholars and integrate current perspectives from a range of European countries. The conference served as a forum to discuss the current status and future perspectives for healthcare professionalism in Europe. Key ideas that emerged during the conference were collected for a joint document which systematises the main insights as formulated by the participants. This position paper, therefore, represents the views of the young generation of European research scientists and healthcare professionals with diverging cultural and scientific backgrounds. In contrast to the ABIM Charter, the position paper is not restricted solely to the medical profession, but encompasses a wide range of occupational groups contributing to contemporary healthcare. The paper summarises the contributors' views on the status quo and future perspectives for healthcare professionalism. Through this, the document can serve as a starting point which highlights topics that need further attention in the debates around professionalism and interprofessionalism in Europe.

The position paper is structured in two parts: Part 1 addresses general characteristics and challenges in contemporary healthcare professionalism, and Part 2 is dedicated to issues of interprofessional cooperation.

Part 1

Healthcare professionalism is characterised by moral rights and duties towards colleagues, patients and society. It is currently challenged by wrong incentive systems and the misuse of professional norms.

- The tenet of medicine to do no harm has remained unchanged since ancient times, although the nature of how this is exercised has changed. The days of paternalistic medicine are over; the focus should now be on an empathetic care in partnership and with respect for the patients' needs.
- Healthcare professionals should be conscious of the fact that the distinctive roles and duties of the different healthcare occupations have been passed on to them historically. A reflective awareness of the historical background is necessary for redefining professions in modern healthcare.
- More autonomy for the healthcare professionals and a stronger involvement in the management of institutions can prove to be beneficial in the long-term. The active engagement of healthcare professionals can reinforce the institutional ethos and bring a higher level of commitment. It enhances healthcare professionals' sense of responsibility for the patients and for their peers.
- In addition to the care for individual patients, healthcare professionals have duties towards the promotion of public health. Some of the greatest contemporary public health needs relate not to the remediation of diseases, but to their prevention. Biomedical enhancement appears to play a tacit and necessary role in public health. If enhancement becomes an increasingly visible part of normal care, this will affect the relation between healthcare professionals and the public.
- Communication constitutes one key aspect of modern healthcare professionalism. Open communication is a prerequisite for holistic and patient-centred care. Next to oral communication, written texts are an important means of healthcare communication. It is crucial to raise awareness among healthcare providers regarding the ethically relevant differences between written and spoken communication.
- Misguided incentive systems pose a challenge to professional conduct in healthcare. Professionalism is, for example, threatened by informal fund collection systems, such as direct payments from patients to physicians. Where these mechanisms are present and tolerated by the system, this provokes a change in the physicians' profile and fosters an orientation toward profit rather than an attitude of altruism and caring.
- The notion of ethics should not be used as a means for exercising state control over the medical profession. The misuse of healthcare ethics committees, as can be currently observed in transitional post-communist societies, diminishes the internal commitment of professionals to serve their patients' best interests and weakens healthcare professionals' confidence in the power of their professional integrity.

Part 2

Healthcare professionalism necessitates a commitment to inter-professional collaboration and education.

- The medical world is ever enlarging and it is often impossible for a single healthcare provider to have all the knowledge necessary to treat a patient appropriately. Without teamwork and respect, healthcare professionals are unable to achieve the best for those for whom they care. In the event of team conflicts, it must be remembered that the patient's health and needs should be primary considerations in decision–making.
- Effective collaboration in interprofessional healthcare teams improves the quality of information exchange and optimises resource utilisation and patient care outcomes. It reduces the impact of human factors, such as bias and fatigue, and minimises the risk of adverse events for patients. Ethical leadership has a positive influence on team members' attitudes, motivation and desirable behaviour.
- The cooperation between hospital managers and the healthcare profess-ionals is essential for effective strategic decision–making. The professionals' expert knowledge as well as the managers' knowledge about strategic planning and implementation are crucial for the survival of hospitals in an increasingly competitive environment.
- Interprofessional learning is increasingly gaining importance in view of rapidly developing medical technologies and complex healthcare environ-ments. *Learning* as an interprofessional and interdisciplinary team is a pre-requisite for effectively *working* as an interprofessional and interdisciplinary team.

Note

1 The following authors contributed to the content of this position paper and agreed with its final form: Sarah Berger, Andrei Famenka, Kirstin Fragemann, Katharina Fürholzer, Alex McKeown, Stephanie Rüsch, Martina Šendula-Pavelić, Dorina Maria Stănescu, Tetiana Stepurko, Clemens Tangerding, Christopher Yu.

References

ABIM Foundation, 2002. Medical professionalism in the new millennium: a Physician Charter. *Annals of Internal Medicine*, 136(3), pp. 243–6.
ABIM Foundation, 2015. Physician Charter. Available through: <www.abimfoundation. org/Professionalism/Physician-Charter.aspx> [accessed 28 August 2015].

Index

access to healthcare 101–2
akrasia 151
artificial nutrition 113; case examples of 120–21, 152–53; decision-making about 114–20, 122–23
authority 139–41, 146, 153–56; challenging 157; *see also* hierarchy

Belarus: misuse of clinical ethics consultation in 89, 93–98; professionalism 89
biomedical citizenship 92
bonuses 82–84; *see also* incentives
brain drain 101–3; effects of 103–5; possible solutions to 106–7

clinical ethics consultation 89, 91–93, 97; in Belarus 93–98
communication 157, 179; decision-making 40–41; hospital managers and 142–43; *see also* physician's letters
communitarianism 103
cosmopolitanism 103
cover-up 83, 157
crew resource management 157
curriculum development 58

decision-making 180; capacity 114–23, 152; challenges to 43–46, 114, 122; collaborative 42–43, 46; education 39–40, 55; ethical leadership in 132–34; hierarchical structures in 41–42, 139, 143–44, 154–59; human resource 82–86; interprofessional 42–43, 113, 118–23, 132; process 118–120; shared 41–42, 55; strategic 144; substituted and supported 114–16, 122; *see also* artificial nutrition
diagnosis-related groups 138

doctor–patient relationship 25; physician's letters in 28–29; implications of medical letters on 30, 32–33; enhancement and 162–63

eating and drinking interventions: *see* artificial nutrition
education: brain drain and 106–7; decision-making 39–40; feedback in 158; interprofessional 39–40, 53–56, 67, 180; pain 53–54, 56–60; postgraduate 57–65, 77–78; undergraduate 54; *see also* teaching
enhancement 163–65, 179: case study of 167–69; distinction between therapy and 166–67; public health 165–66, 169–71
erythropoietin 167–69
ethical leadership 126–27; effects of 127–28, 130–34, 180
ethical values: in ethical leadership 131; *see also* ethical leadership
ethnography 74

Germany 9–22, 29, 53–54, 138–39, 142

healthcare professionals 139–41, 178–80; control over 97–98, 145–46, 179; decision-making by 39–46; increasing need for 102; interprofessional education of 54–56; migration of 101–107; pain management by 52–54, 57, 63–65
healthcare service provision 85, 162–63; ethical behavior in 132–33; in the Ukraine 74, 84–86
healthcare teams 39–43, 54–56, 180: decision-making in 39–46, 113, 118–23; education of 65–67; *see also* interprofessional collaboration

hierarchy 41, 139, 143–44 154–59;
  see also authority
Hippocrates 151
hospital management 138–41, 179–80;
  conflicts with 9, 18–21; in Protestant
  hospitals 14–15; interaction between
  medical staff and 142–46
hospital market 138
Hyder, Adnan A. 93–94, 96

illness prevention 162–63; distinction
  between enhancement and 166–67
incentives 83–84, 143–44, 179;
  see also bonuses
interprofessional collaboration 39–41,
  52–56, 126, 134, 180; decision-
  making in 42–43, 113, 118–23;
  management and 142–146; pain
  management and 52, 55–56; *see also*
  interprofessional decision-making;
  see also interprofessional education;
  see also healthcare teams

medical professionalism 73, 89–91, 133,
  162, 178–80; clinical ethics
  consultation and 89–92, 97–98;
  communication skills and 25, 32–33;
  dealing with the lack of 84;
  enhancement and 163, 169–71;
  political self-concept in 20–22;
  post-Soviet countries and 73–86,
  93–98
Milgram, Stanley 153–56
Mintzberg, Henry 139–141, 142–43,
  145–46
moral deliberation 92
moral duty 102–103, 107, 164, 179
multi-professional teams: *see*
  interprofessional collaboration

Nozick, Robert 103

organisational citizenship behavior
  127–30

pain management 52; interprofessional
  education of 53–54, 56–67
paternalism 115, 163
pathography 31–32
patient autonomy 32–33
patient safety 42–46, 158
percutaneous endoscopic gastrostomy
  113, 152
performance appraisal 81–83

personalised medicine 162
pharmacists 56
physician's letters 25; consequences of
  32–33; content and structure of
  25–26; doctor–patient relationship
  and 28–29; functions and criticism of
  26–28; genre of 31–32; implications
  of 30; teaching 28
post-Soviet countries 73, 84–86, 93–97,
  106; *see also* Belarus; *see also* Ukraine
power distance index 154
professional autonomy 140–141
professional bureaucracy 139–42, 145–46
progressive neurological disease 113,
  152–53; *see also* artificial nutrition
Protestant hospitals 9; self-sacrifice 21;
  motherhouse system in 11–14; 'Third
  way' in 20; withdrawal of 9, 15–17,
  20–21
public health 165, 179; enhancement
  and 163–66, 169–71

quality of health care: chief personnel
  and 142–43; collaborative practice and
  41–46, 54; in the Ukraine 74; stress
  and 151–52

religious institutions in hospital care 12;
  see also Protestant hospitals
right to free movement 102–103, 107

shared decision-making 41–42
sisterhoods 11; *see also* religious
  institutions in hospital care
spoken language 30–31; see also written
  language
strategy making 142–46, 180; role of
  trade unions 17–20; *see also* hospital
  management
Swick, Herbert M. 73, 85–86, 90
system failure 44–46

teaching: brain drain and 104; medical
  letters 25, 28; pain management
  53–54, 56–60; *see also* education
'Third Way' 20

Ukraine 73–74; job appointment in the
  79–81; job appraisal in the 81–83;
  postgraduate education in the 77–78

written language 30–31; *see also* spoken
  language
work attitudes 55, 127–28, 130–31, 180